English for Nurses

—Revised Edition—

by

Margaret Yamanaka

Asahi Press

音声再生アプリ「リスニング・トレーナー」を使った音声ダウンロード

朝日出版社開発のアプリ、「リスニング・トレーナー（リストレ）」を使えば、教科書の音声をスマホ、タブレットに簡単にダウンロードできます。どうぞご活用ください。

◉ アプリ【リスニング・トレーナー】の使い方

《アプリのダウンロード》

App Store または Google Play から「リスニング・トレーナー」のアプリ（無料）をダウンロード

App Storeはこちら▶

Google Playはこちら▶

《アプリの使い方》

① アプリを開き「コンテンツを追加」をタップ
画面上部に【15666】を入力しDoneをタップ

音声ストリーミング配信 》》》

この教科書の音声は、右記ウェブサイトにて無料で配信しています。

https://text.asahipress.com/free/english/

Cover Design: Kenichiro Oshita
Illustration: Maki Watanabe

Introduction

Nursing in Japan continues to change and improve. Along with the increase in foreigners making their home in Japan, is an influx of short stay visitors and tourists. English is not only a language to "study" at school, but also a language to "use" at work in the hospital. From the first day of hospitalization to the day of discharge, this book has the English tools needed for budding nurses in their future jobs.

This book is designed for Japanese students who are now enrolled in a two, three or four year nursing program. Some students will have had one year of college-level English; others may not.

The purpose of this book is twofold; to introduce students to vocabulary they will encounter in doctors' reports and to help students feel competent in situations where they must listen to and speak to foreign patients in English. The aim is to teach students to communicate with patients rather than to give them a fluent command of English.

Each lesson contains a short list of key expressions divided into nurses' expressions and patients' expressions, speaking practice and writing practice, a box of medical vocabulary, and a full dialogue. Speaking practice usually consists of very short dialogues using key expressions or phrases from the longer dialogue. Speaking practice is sometimes preceded by writing practice because some students speak better after they have thought about the words and written them.

Each lesson also contains a communication strategy. Nurses need to communicate with their patients every day, and any techniques they can use to do so are helpful. Amongst the strategies, we encourage students to use their hands to point as well as using other body language, to use compact verbal responses, and other techniques to communicate meaning. Role-play is an important teaching technique to encourage use of communication strategies, and many speaking practice exercises call for role-play.

All lessons also contain a section called Word Power, which helps students understand the meaning of words and teaches prefixes or suffixes so that students can recognize the meanings of even unfamiliar medical words.

Each chapter ends with the dialogue in the form of a fill-in-the-blanks listening exercise. However, by this stage, many students will already be able to estimate what terms are necessary to complete the dialogue.

Finally, it is our hope that students can use this book, not only as an in-class text, but also as a reference when on the ward.

The following people have been very helpful in making this Revised Edition:
Dr. Hideki Kitagawa, Kitagawa Orthopedic Clinic; Dr. Kazuki Yamanaka, Chuno Kosei Hospital; Ms. Alexandra Burke, Ibi Department of Education; Ms. Annette Booth, Prince Charles Hospital; Ms. Julie Meikle, ENAP, Queensland Health; your assistance has been invaluable.

Patricia Parker (First Edition co-author)
Margaret Yamanaka

はしがき

日本の医療現場は変わりつつあります。外国人の入国が増えたり、海外育ちの日本人の帰国が年々増える傾向が見られます。これに伴って多くの臨床医は患者のカルテを書くときに英語を使うようになり、看護師のための特殊な英語教育の必要性が出てきました。

本書は大学・短期大学・専門学校の看護教育を受けている学生を対象に書かれているものです。しかし、学年の指定はありません。

本書の目的は2つです。1、外国人患者に的確な対応ができるようにし、2、カルテに書かれている英語の語彙に触れさせる。本書の狙いは、ナースが流暢な英語を身につけるというよりも、スムーズに患者さんとのコミュニケーションが図れるようにするところにあります。

各レッスンは、次のように構成されています。
☆ key expressions　必須表現（ナースの言葉・患者の言葉）
☆ speaking practice　スピーキングエクササイズ
☆ writing practice　ライティングエクササイズ
☆ medical vocabulary box　医学語彙リスト
☆ dialog ダイアログ。
スピーキングエクササイズは、ダイアログや必須表現にある語句の練習の場となります。場合によって、スピーキングの前に考えをまとめるために、ライティングエクササイズがあります。

各レッスンには communication strategy（コミュニケーションの作戦・方法）があります。患者さんとのコミュニケーションはナースの大事な仕事の一つですので、患者さんを安心させ、上手に扱うためには、様々な工夫が必要です。このセクションではジェスチャー、あいづち、などの工夫を教え、使うように薦めています。また、このような工夫が身に付くようにロールプレイングのエクササイズを増やしています。

各章に Word Power（ワードパワー）のセクションがあります。ここで、よく目にする特殊な医学用語のラテン語やギリシア語の起源を学ぶことによって、新しい言葉に出会ったときに苦労しないようにしています。

各章の終わりに、ディクテーションエクササイズとしてダイアログがあります。しかし、この段階では殆どの学生が、もうどのような言葉がふさわしいのか分かるでしょう。

最後に、本書は授業内の教材としてだけではなく、医療現場での参考本・手引きとしてもお使いいただければ幸いです。

著者

TABLE OF CONTENTS

Introduction / はしがき

Unit 1   Is this your first visit to this hospital?

When a patient enters a hospital or clinic for the first time, the clerk or nurse on duty needs information about the new client. What questions do you think will be asked at first?（初めて病院にかかる人にどんな質問をしますか？）

KEY EXPRESSIONS

NURSES' KEY EXPRESSIONS

1. May I help you?
   「お困りですか？」
2. Is this your first visit to this hospital?
   「この病院に来るのは初めてですか？」
3. Please register over there.
   「あちらで受付をしてください」
4. Please fill in this form.
   「こちらの用紙に記入をお願いします」
5. What is your date of birth?
   「生年月日はいつですか？」

PATIENTS' KEY EXPRESSIONS

1. My name is Hudson, H-U-D-S-O-N.
   「私の名前はハドソン、H-U-D-S-O-N です」
2. I live in Minokamo.
   「私は美濃加茂市に住んでいます」
3. My phone number is (area code 0574) 276-2589.
   「電話番号は、（市外局番 0574）276-2589 です」
4. My date of birth is 16th June, 1983.
   「生年月日は、1983 年の 6 月 16 日です」
5. I work in a factory.
   「私は工場で働いています」

● Initial questions

Some questions can be asked in different ways. Choose a way that suits your needs and is easy to say. （違う風に質問することもできます。自分の必要に応じた表現、また言い易い表現を選びましょう。）

◆ Name

☐ May I ask your name?

☐ Can I have your name please?

☐ What's your name, please?

> **Cultural Quip**
>
> **First name** = Christian name = Given name;　**Middle name**;
> **Last name** = Surname = Family name
>
> eg. Yvonne Maria Christina Alberta Milton
> （middle name が二つ以上ある人がいます。）
>
> eg. Charles Hudson V
> (the fifth generation of eldest sons all named Charles Hudson ハドソン家の長男はチヤールズという名前でその五代目を表します。)
>
> eg. Peter Smythe Sr（senior＝父）& Peter Smythe Jr（junior＝息子）

◆ Address

☐ What is your address?

☐ Where do you live?

☐ Where are you living now?

> **Cultural Quip**
>
> eg. My address is Room 301, Ando Mansion, 46 Honmachi-dori, Minokamo City.
> （住所を言う時は日本語と逆の順番で言う。美濃加茂市本町通り46番地アンドウマンション301号）
>
> eg. I'm sorry, I don't know the address of my hotel.
> I'm staying at the City Hotel.
> （短期間滞在の外国人はホテルの名前しかわからないことがあります。）

◆ Phone Number

☐ What's your telephone number? (cell phone / mobile phone)

☐ May I have a contact number?

☐ Who should we contact in case of an emergency?

◆ Date of Birth (DOB)

☐ What is your date of birth?

　※ When were you born? の場合は主に生まれた年を , When is your
　　birthday? の場合は主に生まれた月日を聞いている。

◆ Occupation

☐ What do you do? / What do you do for a living?

☐ What is your occupation?

☐ What kind of work do you do?

　※ 答えとして I'm a truck driver. でも I drive a truck. でも可能。

◆ Nationality

☐ What is your nationality?

☐ Where do you come from?

　　⇒ Where do you come from originally?

◆ Marital Status

☐ What is your marital status?

☐ Do you have a partner?

☐ Are you married? or single?

> **Cultural Quip**
>
> 答えには married, single, widowed（未亡人）, divorced（離婚者）,
> separated（別居中）, de facto（内縁の妻・夫）があります。国によっ
> て妻・夫別姓もあり、その子供の姓に妻側と夫側のどちらかを選ぶこ
> とができます。又、場合によって、夫人は両方の名を使うこともあり
> ます。
> eg. Mrs. Tanaka-Smit

◆ Dependants*

☐ Do you have any children?

☐ Do you have any dependants?

* Dependants: 扶養家族

■■■ Communication Strategy ■■■
–Asking to repeat information–

As nurses, your duties include passing information between the patient and the doctor. Accuracy is important. Use these phrases when you can't hear, or couldn't fully understand. （ナースの仕事の一部は患者と主治医のつなぎ役であるため、正確さが大切です。患者さんの言葉が分からない、または聞き取れないとき、次のフレーズを使いましょう。）

- ☐ Sorry?
- ☐ Pardon?
- ☐ Please repeat that.
- ☐ Could you say that again?
- ☐ Please speak up.
- ☐ Could you speak more slowly, please?
- ☐ Could you write that down?
- ☐ How do you spell that?
- ☐ Do you mean ...?
- ☐ Did you say (a) or (b)?

● Other questions

Depending on the situation, you may need to ask other questions. Some may be to get important information. Some questions may just be to continue a conversation or to relax a nervous patient. （場合によって、新しい質問を聞かなければいけないときがあります。下記にある文は情報収集のためのものや、緊張した患者さんの気持ちを和らげるための質問です。）

☐ Do you have any brothers or sisters?	自分以外の兄弟は何人いますか？
☐ Are you living with your in-laws?	お舅さんやお姑さんと同居していますか？
☐ What do you do in your spare time?	時間が空いた時は何をしてますか？
☐ What are you interested in?	どういうものに興味を持っていますか？
☐ Do you have any hobbies?	趣味は何ですか？
☐ How long have you been living in Japan?	日本に来て何年ですか？
☐ Have you always lived in this town?	ずっとこの町に住んでいますか？

SPEAKING PRACTICE

Use the above expressions and make out information cards of your patients.

My card

Name: _____

Address: _____

_____

Phone: # _____

DOB: _____

Age: _____

Occupation: _____

Nationality: _____

Marital Status: _____

Patient card

Name: _____

Address: _____

_____

Phone: # _____

DOB: _____

Age: _____

Occupation: _____

Nationality: _____

Marital Status: _____

Patient card

Name: _____

Address: _____

_____

Phone: # _____

DOB: _____

Age: _____

Occupation: _____

Nationality: _____

Marital Status: _____

 WORD POWER

Sometimes, by pulling words apart and looking at word roots and affixes, we can perhaps get a clue to understanding other words. （医学の専門用語の多くはギリシャ・ラテン語に語源を持つ言葉なので、単語を分割して、意味を取れば、他の言葉の意味を理解する手助けにもなります。）

AFFIX	MEANING	EXAMPLES
uni / mono	1 の	union, unilateral, monochrome, monoplegia
bi / di / du	2 の	biannual, biceps, dioxide, duplicate, duodenum
tri / ter	3 の	triplets, triangle, tertiary, triceps, trimester
quad / quart / tetra	4 の	quadrant, quadriceps, quarantine, tetradactyl
quint / penta	5 の	quintuplets, pentose, pentagon

WRITING PRACTICE

Study the words in the Word Power list and find the meanings of the words underlined in the following sentences.（上記の語源のリストを見て、下記の文章中の下線の言葉の意味を a ～ e から選びなさい。）

1. ____ Because of Tom's <u>unilateral</u> facial paralysis, he always seemed to look angry.

2. ____ Studies suggest that <u>biennial</u> breast cancer screening after age 65 reduces the mortality rate of older women.

3. ____ Open heart surgery and other extreme conditions are best treated at <u>tertiary</u> care facilities.

4. ____ As COVID-19 began to spread, people who thought they may have been exposed were told to self-<u>quarantine</u>.

5. ____ The identical Dionne <u>quintuplets</u> born in Canada in 1934 are the first set of quintuplets to survive beyond infanthood.

....

    a. once every two years
    b. five babies
    c. originally 40 days of waiting, any period of separation or isolation
    d. one sided
    e. third level, worst stage (illness), a specialist institution (hospital)

 Mini-Dictionary:

- facial paralysis　顔面神経麻痺
- breast cancer　乳がん
- mortality rate　死亡率
- open heart surgery　開心術
- expose　さらす
- survive　生残る

DIALOGUE 1

First, listen to the recording. Then listen again, and fill in the blanks.（最初は本を見ないで聞きなさい。次に本を見ながら聞いて、空欄を埋めてください。）

● *At the Information Desk:*

Nurse: May I help you?

Patient: Yes, I have a pain in my back and I need to see a doctor.

Nurse: Is this your (1)_____ to this hospital?

Patient: Yes, it is.

Nurse: Then please go to the Registration Desk. It's over there, at Window Number One. There you can get a (2)_____ _____. Then you can see a doctor.

Patient: Thank you.

● *At the Registration Desk:*

Nurse: Please (3)_____ this Registration Form.

Patient: I'm sorry. I can't read Japanese.

Nurse: All right. I'll ask you the questions. First, (4)_____ your name, please?

Patient: Sure. I'm Julia Dennison.

Nurse: (5)_____ that?

Patient: Julia. J-U-L-I-A. and Dennison. That's D-E-N-N-I-S-O-N.

Nurse: And (6)_____?

Patient: You mean in Japan? or back home?

Nurse: In Japan.

Patient: My address is Room 401, 2-6 Senda-machi, Naka-ku, Hiroshima.

Nurse: And (7)_____, please?

Patient: 082-221-8732.

Nurse: What is (8)_____?

Patient: November 16, 1995.

Nurse: And what is (9)_____, please?

Patient: I'm an English teacher.

Nurse: Do you have Japanese National (10)_____?

Patient: Yes. Here is my card.

Nurse: Thank you.

Unit 2　What's the matter?

Before suggesting which department the client should be referred to, we need to find out exactly what the problem is.（患者さんをどの診察科に行かせれば良いのかを決めるため、痛みなどの症状を聞かなければなりません。）

KEY EXPRESSIONS

NURSES' KEY EXPRESSIONS

1. What's the matter?「どうかしましたか？」
2. Where is the pain?「どこが痛いですか？」

*患者さんの症状の尋ね方には、他に次のような言い方もあります。

What's the problem? / What's wrong? / How can I help you?
「どうかしましたか？」

How are you feeling today?
「今日の具合はいかがですか？」

What's brought you here today?
「今日はどうされましたか？」

Hello, Mrs. Green. What's the trouble?
「グリーンさん、こんにちは。どうかしましたか？」

PATIENTS' KEY EXPRESSIONS

1. I feel sick.「気持ちが悪いです」
2. I have a headache.〈名詞＋ ache〉「頭痛がします」＊
3. I have sore eyes.〈形容詞＋名詞〉「眼が痛いです」
4. My throat hurts.〈名詞＋動詞〉「のどが痛いです」

＊頭（head）、耳（ear）、胃（stomach）、背（back）、歯（tooth）のみに使います。

＊痛む場所が広い場合、"pain" を使って、"I have a pain in my 〜" と言います）

I have a pain in my leg.
「足が痛いです」

When you ask a question, or a patient tells you her problem, always *look at the person* you are talking with. Also, wherever appropriate, *use the patient's name*. (患者さんと話すとき、患者さんの顔を見て話してください。直接目を見るのが苦手ならば、おでこでもあごでもいいです。そして、状況に応じて、患者さんの名前を使ってください。)

> How are you feeling today, Mrs.Green?

WRITING PRACTICE 1

Label the parts of the body pictured below. (体の各部分を英語で書いてください。)

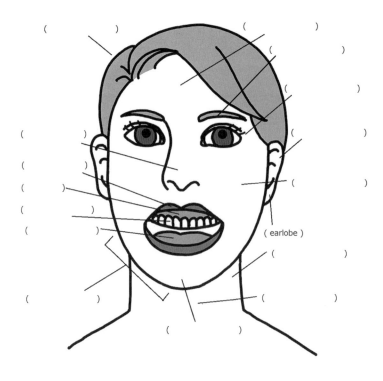

(earlobe)

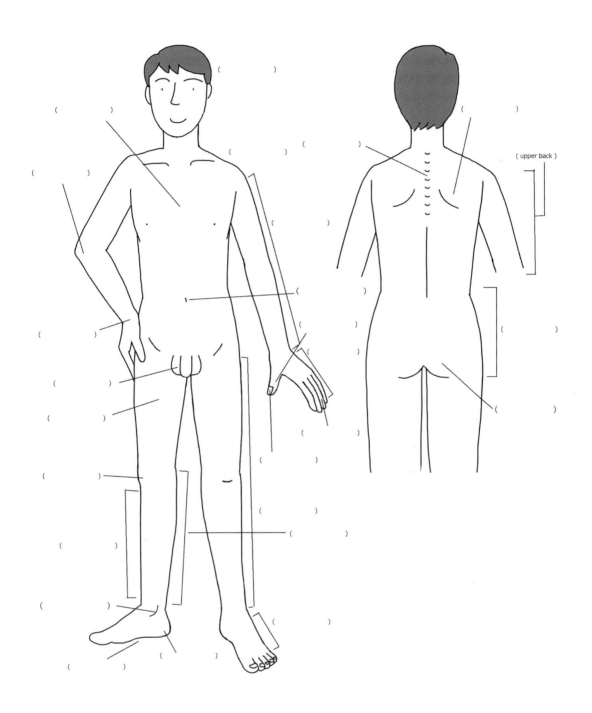

(upper back)

Now check your work with the Vocabulary list on the next page.
（次のページの語彙リストでチェックしてください。）

MEDICAL VOCABULARY
–Parts of the Body–

【頭部・顔・首】

hair	髪	head	頭	forehead	額
ear	耳	neck	首	face	顔
eyebrow	眉	eye	眼	eyelashes	睫
cheek	頬	nose	鼻	mouth	口
lips	唇	tooth	歯	gums	歯茎
tongue	舌	chin	顎先	jaw	顎

【胴体】

chest	胸	breast	胸／乳房	lower back	腰
waist	腰（のくびれ）	shoulder	肩	back	背中
abdomen	腹部	buttocks	臀部	genitals	生殖器
spine	背骨	shoulder blade	肩甲骨		

【四肢】

hand	手	fingers	指	thumb	親指
palm	掌	nail	爪	elbow	肘
arm	腕	wrist	手首	leg	脚
foot	足	thigh	太腿	knee	膝
shin	脛	calf	脹脛	ankle	足首
heel	踵	toes	足の指	sole	足の裏

【その他】

throat	喉	tonsils	扁桃	bones	骨
veins	静脈	stomach	胃	muscles	筋肉
arteries	動脈	ligament	靭帯	joints	関節
ribs	肋骨	pelvis	骨盤	hipbone	寛骨（かんこつ）

((🔊)) SPEAKING PRACTICE

Practice the following dialogues with your partner. Remember the Communication Strategy above, and look at your partner when you are asking a question.（質問をする時相手を見ながら、会話の練習をしましょう。）

① **名詞：**   I have a 〜 ache.（頭、耳、胃、背、歯　のみ）
22
　　　　　　 N: May I help you?
　　　　　　 P: Yes. I have a bad <u>head</u>ache.
　　　　　　 N: I see. Please wait here until your name is called.

① **形容詞＋：** I have a sore 〜 . I have sore 〜 s.
23
　　　　　　 N: What's the matter?
　　　　　　 P: I have a sore <u>shoulder</u>.
　　　　　　 N: I see. The doctor will see you shortly.

① **＋動詞：** My 〜 hurts. My 〜 s hurt.
24
　　　　　　 P: I need to see a doctor.
　　　　　　 N: What's the matter?
　　　　　　 P: My <u>neck</u> hurts.

① 痛む場所が広ければ "pain" を用いて：I have a pain in my 〜 .
25
　　　　　　 N: May I help you?
　　　　　　 P: I have a pain in my <u>leg</u>.
　　　　　　 N: Where exactly is the pain?
　　　　　　 P: Here.

● Now substitute other parts of the body for the underlined words.（他の体の部分を入れ替えて練習しましょう。）

〜 ache:	a) 胃	b) 耳	c) 背
a sore 〜 :	a) 指	b) 眼	c) 足首
My 〜 hurts:	a) 手	b) 膝	c) 喉
a pain in my 〜 :	a) 腕	b) 大腿	c) 胸

WRITING PRACTICE 2

Read and understand what symptoms the patient is complaining of.
（患者さんが話した症状を理解し、記録しましょう。）

Pt (A): "I have a sore leg. My knee hurts, too."
Record: *The patient has pain in their leg and knee.*
又は、日本語で「患者は、脚と膝が痛い」

Pt (B): "I have a terrible earache. It's my left ear that's sore."
Record: *The patient has pain in their left ear.*
又は、日本語で「患者は左の耳が痛い」

Pt 1: "My throat hurts, and I'm a bit feverish."

_____

Pt 2: "My wrist is sore. And so is the base of my thumb."

_____

Pt 3: "I have a pain in my chest, especially when I cough or sneeze."

_____

Pt 4: "I have a sore back. Especially around the base of my spine."

_____

Pt 5: "It's my eyes. There's flashes of light and lots of flecks floating around."

_____

WORD POWER

AFFIX	MEANING	EXAMPLES
man / mani	手	manipulate, manicure, manage, maintain
cap / capit	頭	caput, per capita, capitate bone, capitular joint
dent	歯	dental care, orthodontic, dentures, dentist
ped	足	pedicure, pedestrian, impede, pedal
corp	体	corpulent, corpuscle, corpus, corpse

WRITING PRACTICE 3

Study the words in the Word Power list and find the meanings of the words underlined in the following sentences.（前ページの語源リストを見て、下記の文章中の下線の言葉の意味を a ～ e から選びなさい。）

1. ＿＿＿ The estimated <u>per capita</u> consumption of fish in 2015 was 50.8kg in Japan, and as little as 6.8kg in the U.S.

2. ＿＿＿ White <u>corpuscles</u> are an important part of the body's defense system.

3. ＿＿＿ Tell Mr. Green to take out his <u>dentures</u> before the operation.

4. ＿＿＿ The ambulance has just brought in a man who was hit by a car while crossing a <u>pedestrian</u> crossing.

5. ＿＿＿ Mrs. Arai asked for a <u>manicure</u> before her grandchildren came to visit.

a. care of hands, fingers, or fingernails
b. false teeth
c. a small round body mass; eg. blood cell
d. by head; for each person
e. someone who travels on foot

 Mini-Dictionary:

- consumption　消費
- grandchildren　孫
- ambulance　救急車
- operation　手術

DIALOGUE 2

First, listen to the recording. Then listen again, and fill in the blanks.

N: Good morning, Mr. Jones.

P: Good morning.

N: (1)_____?

P: Well, I was working in the garden the other day...

N: Yes?

P: ...and (2)_____.

N: (3)_____. I'm sorry. Dr. Suzuki

isn't (4)_____ today.

P: Dr. Suzuki always looks at (5)_____,

doesn't he?

N: Yes. You usually see Dr. Suzuki.

P: Who can I see today?

N: First, (6)_____ is the pain?

P: Here.

N: I see. You have (7)_____.

P: Yes.

N: Do you have (8)_____?

P: Oh yes. (9)_____, here.

N: Ok, Mr. Jones. Can you just sit down over there? Your name

(10)_____.

Unit 3　You need to see a Dermatologist.

WARM-UP

When a client enters a clinic or hospital, the nurse needs to know what medical problem brings them to the doctor.　If the client is in a lot of pain, he or she（又は "they"）needs to see a doctor immediately.（場合によっては、患者さんが病院に来た時に緊急かどうかを把握する必要があります。また、欧米では、一般外来にかからず最初からスピーディに診てもらえる ICU クリニックに行く人もいます。）

KEY EXPRESSIONS

NURSES' KEY EXPRESSIONS

1. Do you have any other symptoms?
   「他に症状はありますか？」
2. How long have you had the pain?
   「痛みはどのくらい続いていますか？」
3. You need to see a Dermatologist.
   「皮膚科医に診てもらう必要があります」

PATIENTS' KEY EXPRESSIONS

1. I have a rash. It's itchy.
   「発疹があります。痒いです」
2. I was stung by a wasp. My hand is swollen.
   「ハチに刺されました。手が腫れています」
3. I feel dizzy.
   「めまいがします」
4. I feel nauseous.
   「吐き気がします」
5. I have a fever.
   「熱があります」

■■■ Communication Strategy ■■■
–Ask specific questions–

When a patient tells you her problem, she may be too upset to give the details you need. By *asking several specific questions* you can lead the patient into giving you the information you need. This rapport also helps patient-nurse relations. （痛みが激しい場合、患者さんが興奮して十分な情報をくれない場合もあります。質問が適切であればコミュニケーションが良くなり、必要な情報もよりよいものになります。）

P: I think I have a cold.
N: Do you have a fever?
P: Yes.
N: Do you have any other symptoms?
P: Yes. I have a runny nose.

SPEAKING PRACTICE 1

Make conversations using the strategies and expressions you have learnt. Then substitute the underlined words with other phrases below.
（以下の会話例を練習し、下線部を入れ替えて、練習を続けてください。）

N: What's the matter?

P: <u>My throat hurts</u>.[a]

N: I see. Do you have any other symptoms?

P: I have <u>a bad cough</u>.[b]

N: How long have you had this problem?

P: <u>For three days</u>.[c]

....

	(a)	(b)	(c)
1.	"My knee hurts	/ a swollen leg	/ for about a week"
2.	"I have a fever	/ a runny nose	/ for 2 days"
3.	"My face is itchy	/ red pimples	/ for 3 days"
4.	"I have sore eyes	/ a headache	/ on and off for about a month"

WRITING PRACTICE 1

Continue the previous exercise with other students, asking if the patient has any other symptoms. Record the patient's symptoms（症状）and their duration（期間）.

	Pt Name	Symptoms	Duration
eg	*Yoshio*	*backache, sore shoulders, stiff neck*	*2 weeks*
1			
2			
3			

MEDICAL VOCABULARY
– Departments –

- Cardiology　　　　　　循環器科　　　Cardiologist
  　　　　　　　　　　　　　　　　　　　※ Heart Surgeon 心臓外科医

- Dentistry　　　　　　　歯科　　　　　Dentist
- Dermatology　　　　　　皮膚科　　　　Dermatologist
- Endocrinology　　　　　内分泌内科　　Endocrinologist
- Gynaecology（Gynecology）婦人科　　　　Gynaecologist
- Gastroenterology　　　　消化器内科　　Gastroenterologist
- Internal Medicine　　　　内科　　　　　Internist
- Neurology　　　　　　（脳）神経科　　Neurologist
- Obstetrics　　　　　　　産科　　　　　Obstetrician
  　　※ Obstetrics and Gynecology are often combined, to become "Ob-gyn"［オブジン］.

- Ophthalmology = Eye Specialist　眼科　　Ophthalmologist
- Orthopaedics（Orthopedics）整形外科　Orthopaedist
- Otorhinolaryngology　　耳鼻咽喉科　　Otolaryngologist
  　　　　　　　　　　　　　　　　　　　= (ENT) Ears, Nose, and
  　　　　　　　　　　　　　　　　　　　　 Throat Specialist

- Paediatrics（Pediatrics）小児科　　　Pediatrician
- Psychiatry　　　　　　　精神科　　　　Psychiatrist
- Radiology　　　　　　　放射線科　　　Radiologist
  　　※ 海外では Medical Imaging が一般的でレントゲン以外に CT、MRI、超音波診断などを行う。
  　　　病院やクリニックの外にある場合もあり、名前に Imaging がついていることがよくある。

- Rehabilitation　　　　　リハビリ　　　Therapist
  （Physiotherapy, Occupational Therapy, Speech Therapy）
- Surgery　　　　　　　　外科　　　　　Surgeon
  　　※ In England and Australia, many doctors (General Practiners) run their own clinics and
  　　　often use "Surgery" in the name.

Unit 3　You need to go to Dermatology.

Other Hospital Departments / Wards

● Maternity Ward (Antenatal Clinic)	産科病棟	Midwife
● Plastic Surgery	形成外科	Plastic Surgeon
● Intensive Care Unit (ICU) (NICU Neonatal Intensive Care Unit)	集中治療部 (新生児集中治療室)	
● Oncology	腫瘍学	Oncologist
● Outpatient's	外来	Doctor (G.P.)

※ 海外では患者はまず Outpatient's に行き、後に専門医に紹介される。

● Pathology	病理学	Pathologist

※ In England and Australia, patients will go to Pathology to have blood tests, etc. done.

● Pharmacy	薬局	Pharmacist
● Urology	泌尿器科	Urologist

WRITING PRACTICE 2

Review the 5 "ache" words and suggest which department the patient should go to. ("ache" は体の5つの部分、頭・耳・歯・胃・背中だけに使われます)

Eg.　The patient has a toothache.
　　　What department does they need to go to?
　　　They need to go to Dentistry.

1. The patient has a headache.
   What department does he need to go to?

   _____

2. The patient has a stomachache.
   What department does he need to go to?

   _____

3. The patient has a backache.
   Who does she need to see?

   _____

4. The patient has an earache.
   Who does she need to see?

   _____

WORD POWER

Note that many words for medical departments end in -ology. That is a suffix meaning "study of." （単語を分解し、語源が分かれば、新しい言葉の意味も分かるようになります。例えば -ology の付いている単語は「〜学」という意味だと分かれば、病院内の各専門のほとんどが分かります。）

The following affixes will help you understand other medical vocabulary:

AFFIX	MEANING	EXAMPLES
derm	皮膚	dermatology, dermatitis
neuro	神経	neurology, neurochemistry
ortho	真っすぐな・正常な	orthopedics, orthodontics
radio	放射線・熱・光	radiology, radiation, radiotherapy
cardio	心臓	cardiology, electrocardiograph

 # WRITING PRACTICE 3

Study the affixes in the Word Power list and match the meanings with the words underlined in the sentences below. （上記の語源のリストを見て、下記の文章の中の下線の言葉の意味を a 〜 e から探しなさい。）

1. ____ One way for patients suffering from diabetes to take insulin is by <u>hypodermic</u> injections.

2. ____ Doctors tried to clear the cancer with <u>radiotherapy</u>.

3. ____ Jennifer's father died from a <u>cardiac</u> arrest.

4. ____ The patient was given an ointment for her <u>neurodermatosis</u>.

5. ____ After the car accident, Ted had to wear an <u>orthopedic</u> collar for several weeks.

a. heart
b. to straighten, correct
c. under the skin
d. therapy using high energy rays
e. nervous condition involving the skin

 Mini-Dictionary:
- suffer from （病気に）かかる
- insulin インシュリン
- ointment 軟膏
- diabetes 糖尿病
- injection 注射
- accident 事故

Unit 3　You need to go to Dermatology.

SPEAKING PRACTICE 2

Study the model and then, with your partner, make new conversations. （見本となる会話を練習してから、下線文の症状を下のリストの語句を使って入れ替え、患者さんに必要な診察科を提案しましょう。）

N: What's the trouble?

P: <u>My throat hurts</u>. (a)

N: I see. You need to go to the <u>ENT</u> (Ears, Nose & Throat) Department.

P: Where is it?

N: I'll take you there.

Substitute the symptom (a) with the ones below. Then advice the patient as to which department they should go.

Pt.1. "I have sore eyes. There was crust on my eyelids this morning."

Pt.2. "I cut my finger."

Pt.3. "I have a very painful shoulder."

Pt.4. "My child has a fever."

Pt.5. "I fell down playing tennis. My ankle is swollen."

Pt.6. "I seem to be sneezing all the time."

Pt.7. "I've got heartburn."

SPEAKING PRACTICE 3

Practice the following model and then substitute other body parts and departments for the underlined words. Use items from List (A) & (B) below. For item (C), use your knowledge to decide.（患者さんの症状を下のリストに沿って入れ替え、ペアで会話を練習しなさい。）

N: May I help you?

P: Yes. (A)<u>My child is sick</u>.

N: I'm sorry to hear that. What exactly is the problem?

P: (B)<u>He has an extremly high fever</u>.

N: Is this an emergency?

P: I hope he* can be seen to as quickly as possible.

N: You need to go to the (C)<u>Pediatrics</u> Department. I'll show you where to go.

(* he / she / I を適切に)

Pt.1. (A)"I don't feel well."　(B)"I'm having trouble breathing.

Pt.2. "I had an accident."　"I spilt hot oil over my fingers."

Pt.3. "My mother is sick."　"She suddenly became dizzy and fell."

Pt.4. "I think I have the flu."　"I have a stuffy nose and aching muscles."

Pt.5. "I need a doctor."　"I have a painful rash on my chest."

> **Cultural Quip**
>
> In some parts of the United States, because of the long waiting time at regular clinics, more and more regular patients are going to the Emergency Section, in the hope that they will be served quickly. Therefore, this question is regularly asked in some hospitals. （最近のアメリカでは、一般の診療場で待つ時間が長いため、多くの外来患者はより早く診てもらえる救急セクションにかかるので、日常的に「緊急ですか」と質問するようになった。）

DIALOGUE 3

First, listen to the recording. Then listen again, and fill in the blanks.

Nurse: Hello, Mrs. McKenna. (1)_____
today?

Patient: I'd like to see the doctor, please.

Nurse: Is this (2)_____?

Patient: No, I don't think so.

Nurse: What's the matter?

Patient: I have (3)_____.

Nurse: A rash on your back? (4)_____?

Patient: Yes, it's very itchy.

Nurse: I see. (5)_____ have you had the rash?

Patient: About three or four days.

Nurse: I see. Are there any other problems? Do you (6)_____

_____?

Patient: No. I don't think I have a fever.

Nurse: Have you been (7)_____ lately, Mrs.
McKenna?

Patient: Oh. Well. I'm not sure. Perhaps it's (8)_____,
but I thought I should have a doctor check it.

Nurse: Yes, it's a good idea for a doctor to check it. You need to go to
the (9)_____. Nurse Saito will take
you there.

Patient: Thank you.

Nurse Saito: Hello, Mrs. McKenna. Please, (10)_____.

Unit 4　Let me direct you to Radiology.

Hospitals can sometimes seem like a maze（迷路）to patients. If asked by a visitor, could you explain how to get to your classroom from the front entrance of your school? Giving good, easy to follow directions is also part of good communication.（病院は知らない人にとって迷路みたいなものです。病院を訪れた人に行き先の案内ができるようになりましょう。）

KEY EXPRESSIONS

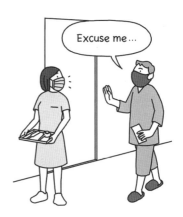

Excuse me…

NURSES' KEY EXPRESSIONS

1. Take the elevator up to the 2nd floor.
   「エレベータで2階に上がってください」
2. Go downstairs to Radiology.
   「階段を降りて放射線科に行ってください」
3. Go straight along the hall.
   「廊下をまっすぐ進んでください」
4. Turn right at the end of the hall.
   「廊下の突き当たりを右に曲がってください」
5. Dermatology is on the left.
   「皮膚科は左にあります」

PATIENTS' KEY EXPRESSIONS

1. Where is Radiology?
   「放射線科はどこにありますか？」
2. Can you tell me how to get to Radiology?
   「放射線科への行き方を教えてください」
3. Where do I go to get an X-ray?
   「レントゲン検査を受けるにはどこに行けばいいですか？」

■■■ Communication Strategy ■■■
–Shadowing–

When you are listening, listen actively. We can *shadow* the speaker by repeating key words or phrases he or she has said. ("Shadowing" は相手の言ったことを繰り返すことです。)

For example:

A: How do I get from here to the lounge?

B: Go straight. At the first corner turn right. You'll see the elevators.

A: *Turn right* and I'll *see the elevators*?

B: Yes. Take the elevator to the third floor.

A: *Third floor*.

B: Get out of the elevator and turn left. You'll see the lounge area on the right, just past the stairs.

A: *Turn left* and I'll see it *on the right*?

B: Yes.

Cultural Quip

Foreigners with sick spouses, children, or other relatives, may also ask for directions to a nearby church or mosque, an international phone box, or a bank that handles foreign money or an A.T.M. Be sure to know where these places are as soon as you move to a new hospital. (外国人に聞かれたときに、病院の近くの教会や国際電話のボックスなどがどこにあるか答えられると良いですね。)

"Go ～" と "It's ～" を使って、患者さんを適切に目的地まで案内しましょう。

"Go that way. It's next to the Kiosk."
「あちらに行ってください。キオスクの隣にあります」

VOCABULARY FOR GIVING DIRECTIONS

next to / beside

between A and B

(○) in front of

(○) behind / in back of (米)

across from / opposite

straight along

past

(○) around the corner (from□)

(○) on the left / (□) on the right

the third door on the left

(○) turn left / (□) turn right

(at) the end of the hall (corridor)

WRITING PRACTICE 1

Describe where the following things are in your school building. (以下の物が あなたの学校の周辺でどこにあるかを説明してみましょう。)

1. Where is the nearest vending machine?

   _____

2. Give directions to a cafeteria, or a nice place to sit and talk.

   _____

WRITING PRACTICE 2

Use the map below and continue to answer the questions. Begin from the Information Desk.（下記の地図を使って、インフォメーション・カウンターから患者さんの案内を続けましょう。）

1. Where is Ophthalmology?

   Go upstairs...

2. Can you tell me how to get to Rehabilitation?

   Go that way.

3. How can I get to Neurology?

   Go straight along here.

4. Where are the toilets?

   Go that way.

● Here is a map of Chuo Hospital, 1st and 2nd floors.

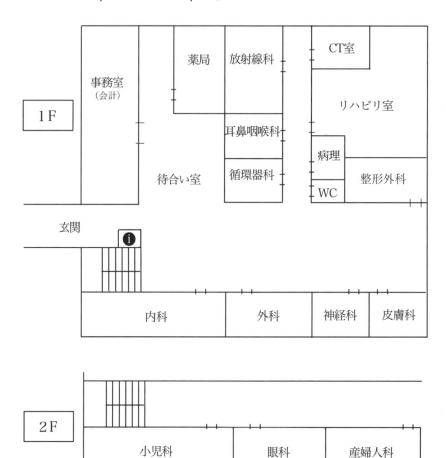

((⬤ SPEAKING PRACTICE

Using the map of Chuo Hospital and the list of names of medical departments, help the patient as they go around to various departments.

Use phrases like these:

P: Where is _____? 又は

How do I get to the _____ Department? など

N: It's next to _____, on the right. 又は

It's around the corner from _____. など

....

① 総合案内 → 小児科 _____

② 小児科 → 耳鼻科 _____

③ 耳鼻科 → 放射線科 _____

④ 放射線科 → 会計 _____

WRITING PRACTICE 3

Here is a ward floor plan. Complete the conversations below.
（間取り図を見て、会話を完成させましょう。）

						310	309
312	311	Kitchen	E.V.		Toilets	Laundry	308
							307
301	302	303	N.S.		305		306

Mr. Black has arrived at the Orthopedics Ward on the 3rd floor to visit his friend Mr. Green who is a patient in Room 309.

● At Nurses' Station

Mr. Black: Excuse me. My friend, Mr. Green, is in Room 309. Can you tell me how to get there?

Nurse: _____

_____

Unit 4   Let me direct you to Radiology.

● In Room 309

Mr. Black: Hi!

Mr. Green: Hi! I've been waiting for you. Can you make us a cup of tea?

Mr. Black: Sure. Where's the kitchen?

Mr. Green: _____

_____

● In the kitchen

Mr. Black: Excuse me, Nurse. I need to wash some towels. Is there a laundry on this floor?

Nurse: _____

_____

● In the laundry

Mr. Black: Hi, Mr. Brown! Long time no see! Visiting someone?

Mr. Brown: Hi. Yes, I'm here to visit my brother in Room 301.

Mr. Black: Oh, where's that?

Mr. Brown: _____

Mr. Black: Okay, I might see you later then.

Mr. Brown: See you.

● Back in Room 309

Mr. Green: It's been great seeing you. And thanks for all your help.

Mr. Black: No problem. But I'm afraid I really have to go now.

Mr. Green: Oh!?

Mr. Black: But first, could you tell me where the nearest pay-phone is?

Mr. Green: _____

Mr. Black: Good. Thanks. Bye.

Mr. Green: Good-bye.

WORD POWER

AFFIX	MEANING	EXAMPLES
com / con / col	共に	communication, contact, combine, condolence, collect
sub / suf / sup	下に・下から	suffer, support, subject, sublingual, supine
in	中に	insert, inject, incision, infection, intestines
ex	外へ	expel, expire, external, exclude, excretion
pro	先へ	progress, project, protect, prolong, prone

 # WRITING PRACTICE 4

Study the prefixes in the Word Power list and match the meanings with the words underlined in the sentences below. （上記の語源のリストを見て、下記の文章中の下線の言葉の意味を a ～ e から探しなさい。）

1. ___ We need to be careful of different medicine <u>combinations</u>.

2. ___ Modern science allows us to <u>prolong</u> life.

3. ___ Julia's husband allowed the doctor to disconnect her from the life-<u>support</u>ing machines.

4. ___ The surgeon made an <u>incision</u> over the bunion to remove bony growth.

5. ___ Be sure the patient does not swallow any medicine intended for <u>external</u> use.

    a. extend; make longer

    b. cut into

    c. putting two or more things together

    d. outside

    e. assist, carry from under

 Mini-Dictionary:

- allow to　可能にする；許す
- disconnect　はずす
- life-supporting machine　生命維持装置
- bunion　バニオン・腱膜瘤
- bony　骨のような
- swallow　飲み込む
- intended for...　～のために

DIALOGUE 4

First, listen to the recording. Then listen again, and fill in the blanks.

Patient: Excuse me, can you tell me where the elevators are?

Nurse: Sure. (1)_____ down this hall and you'll see them.

Patient: On the right side or the left side?

Nurse: They're (2)_____. What department are you looking for?

Patient: I need to get an x-ray done. The Medical Imaging Department is on the second floor, isn't it?

Nurse: That's right. (3)_____ to the second floor. Get out of the elevator and (4)_____.

Patient: Ah-huh.

Nurse: Go to (5)_____, and the Radiology Department is the (6)_____ _____. It's just past Orthopedics.

Patient: From the elevator, I turn right, go to the end of the hall, and it's on the left?

Nurse: (7)_____.

Patient: Are there any stairs in this building?

Nurse: Yes, the stairway is (8)_____ the elevators.

Patient: Just past the elevators?

Nurse: Yes. You can take the stairs to the second floor if you like. (9) _____ show you the way?

Patient: No, thanks. I think I can find it myself.

Nurse: If you have (10) _____, just ask someone to help you.

Patient: Thank you.

Unit 5　Let's check your height and weight.

WARM-UP

Often the doctor wants the nurse to check the patient's condition before the patient talks to the doctor. What information does the nurse or doctor need about a patient who comes in for a checkup? When you visited the doctor last time, did the nurse ask about your height and weight? （医師の診察の前に看護師は患者さんの体調を確認することがあります。診察の前に医師はどんな情報が必要でしょうか。あなたは病院に行った時、身長と体重を聞かれたことがありますか。）

KEY EXPRESSIONS

NURSES' KEY EXPRESSIONS

1. What is your height? / How tall are you?
   「身長はいくつですか？」
2. What is your weight? / How much do you weigh?
   「体重はどのくらいですか？」
3. Let's check your blood pressure.
   「血圧を測らせてください」
4. Let's check your pulse.
   「脈拍をとらせてください」

PATIENTS' KEY EXPRESSIONS

1. I'm 160 cm tall. / I'm 5 feet 3 inches tall.
   「身長は 160 センチです / 5 フィート 3 インチです」
2. I weigh 150 pounds. / I'm 68 kilograms.
   「体重は 150 ポンドです / 68 キロです」
3. I'm a little overweight.
   「私は少し太り過ぎです」

MEDICAL VOCABULARY
– Measurements –

● **Height** (身長)
1 inch　　= 2.54 centimeters
12 inches = 1 foot
1 foot　　= 30 centimeters
　　　　　　or 0.3 meters

● **Weight** (体重)
1 pound 〈米〉= 453.6 grams
　　　　　　　or 0.45 kilograms
1 stone 〈英〉 = 14 pound (約 6.35kg.)
1 kilogram　= 2.2 pounds

● **Body Temperature** (体温)
C = Centigrade or Celsius　= 摂氏　※ 0° C = 32° F
F = Fahrenheit　　　　　　= 華氏 (アメリカ合衆国でのみ、まだ広く使われている)
　　36.7°C = "thirty-six *point* seven *degrees*" = normal body temperature
　　thermometer = 体温計・温度計
　　fever = 熱 / feverish = 熱っぽい

● **Blood Pressure** (血圧)
170 / 80 = "one hundred seventy *over* eighty"
hypertension = high blood pressure = 高血圧
hypotension = low blood pressure = 低血圧

● **Pulse** (脈)
65 bpm = "sixty-five *beats per minute*"

● **Oxygen Levels** (SpO2) (酸素濃度)
Oxygen saturation in the blood (経皮的動脈血酸素飽和度)
= Pulse Oximetry
(Normal range = 96%-98%)

● **Waist Circumference** (WC) (胴囲周り)
Adiposity Waist Measurement (肥満のウエスト測定)
Place a tape measure horizontally around the abdomen at the top of the hip
bone (iliac crest) (メジャーを腸骨稜の位置にし、胴周りを測る)

● **Fundal Height** (SFH) (子宮底長)
= The distance from the pubic bone (symphysis pubis) to the top of the
　　uterus (uterine fundus); to assess fetal growth and development.
　　(恥骨結合から子宮低の最高点までの長さ)

Cultural Quip

In the U.S., people still give their weight in "pounds", while in England
and Australia, older people may still use "stones". The young usually
use metric measurements. A person of 173cm might say "I'm 1 metre
73." (アメリカ人はよくポンドを使い、年配のイギリス人やオーストラリ
ア人はストーンを使います。173 センチの若者は「1 メートル 73」と説明
するでしょう。)

WRITING PRACTICE 1

Complete the following, using **weigh** or **weight**: **Weigh**（動詞）と **Weight**（名詞）
を使い分けて空欄を埋めなさい。

a. His _____ has been increasing recently.

b. The nurse checked the patient's _____.

c. If you _____ too much, it may affect your general health.

d. Last year she _____ 50 kg., but now she _____
   only 45 kg.

e. Use this scale to _____ all the new patients.

SPEAKING PRACTICE 1

With a classmate, practice asking about your patient's height and weight.
Substitute other words and numbers for the underlined words. Use your
imagination!（とても不健康な人が病院に行ったことにしましょう。大変太ってい
る人。または、ひどくやせている人。いろんな状況を想像して、楽しく練習しましょ
う。）

N: How tall are you?

P: I'm not sure.

N: I'll check your height. Stand up against this scale. You are 160 cm.
    tall.

N: How much do you weigh?

P: I'm not sure.

N: I'll check your weight. Stand on this scale. You weigh 45 kg.

P: Is that normal?

N: You're a little underweight.

Patient Name _____	Patient Name _____
Patient's height: Patient's weight:	Patient's height: Patient's weight:

Unit 5   Let's check your height and weight.

■■■ Communication Strategy ■■■
–Use body language–

Use body language. *Point* as you give directions. Keep a friendly *smile*. If the patient is in pain or under stress, *hold* the patient. *Touch* conveys concern. *Show* sympathy （ボディランゲージを使いましょう。手を使って案内をし、笑顔を保ちましょう。患者さんが苦痛やストレスを感じていたなら、手を握り心配していることを伝えましょう。）

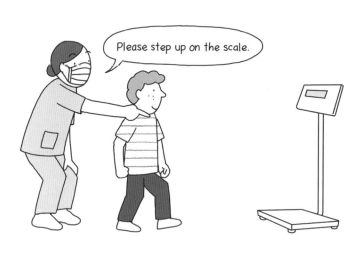

Please step up on the scale.

SPEAKING PRACTICE 2

Check your partner's vital signs (blood pressure, temperature, and pulse). Use real instruments if possible. Use the following models, and record the answers. （できれば本物の器具を使って会話の練習をし、答えを記録しなさい。）

B.P.　N: Let's check your blood pressure. Hold out your arm, and relax.

(Pause.)

N: Your blood pressure is —.

Temp. N: Let's check your temperature. Put this thermometer under your arm, like this.

(Pause.)

N: Your temperature is —.

P: Is that normal?

N: Yes, it is. / It's a little high. / It's a little low.

Pulse N: Let's check your pulse. Let me hold your wrist. Just relax.

(Pause.)

N: Your pulse is —.

SpO2 N: Let's check the oxygen in your blood.
Let me place a sensor on your fingertip.

Patient Name _____	**Patient Name** _____
Patient's B.P.: (Normal / High / Low)	Patient's B.P.: (Normal / High / Low)
Patient's temp.: (Normal / High / Low)	Patient's temp.: (Normal / High / Low)
Pulse: b.p.m. (Normal / High / Low)	Pulse: b.p.m. (Normal / High / Low)
SpO2: % (Normal / Low)	SpO2: % (Normal / Low)

Unit 5   Let's check your height and weight.

WORD POWER

AFFIX	MEANING	EXAMPLES
hyper	超・過度の	hypertension, hyperactive, hyperpnea
hypo	下・過少の	hypotension, hypoglycemia, hypothermia
therm	熱	thermal, thermometer, thermograph
max / magn	最大	maximum, climax, magnify
mini / micro	最小	minimum, minority, microscope

 # WRITING PRACTICE 3

Study the affixes in the Word Power list and match the meanings with the words underlined in the sentences below.（上記の語源のリストを見て、下記の文章中の下線の言葉の意味を a ～ e から探しなさい。）

1. ＿＿ A hyperactive child usually has difficulty sitting still.

2. ＿＿ Use a reliable thermometer, if you suspect that the child has a fever.

3. ＿＿ Hypothermia is sometimes used to help cardiac arrest survivors.

4. ＿＿ For some types of treatments, it may take several weeks to get the maximum effect of the medication.

5. ＿＿ Pamphlets on various medical topics are available for ethnic minority groups in Australia.

....

   a. low (body) temperature

   b. highest

   c. over active

   d. a group much smaller than the average

   e. a measure of (body) heat

 Mini-Dictionary:
- sit still　じっと座っている
- reliable　信頼できる
- suspect　疑う
- treatment　治療
- ethnic　人種

DIALOGUE 5

First, listen to the recording. Then listen again, and fill in the blanks.

Nurse: What is (1)_____?

Patient: I'm six foot two inches.

Nurse: What is (2)_____?

Patient: I weigh a hundred and ninety pounds.

Nurse: How many kilograms is that?

Patient: I don't know. Sorry.

Nurse: OK. Let's check your weight. Please take off your shoes and stand here, (3)_____.

          [pause]   Your weight is 86 kg.

Patient: I'm (4)_____.

Nurse: Now let's check your height. Stand still. A sliding bar will touch the top of your head.

          [pause] Your height is 188 cm. The machine shows that your BMI is 24.3. That's just within the (5)_____, but you're very close to being overweight.

          Next let's (6) _____. Put this

          thermometer (7) _____, like this.

          [pause]   Your temperature is 36.8 degrees Centigrade.

Patient: Do I have a fever?

Nurse: No, your temperature is normal.

          And now let's (8)_____. Hold out your arm, and relax.

          [pause] Your blood pressure is (9)_____.

          Do you usually (10)_____?

Patient: No, I don't. Maybe it's a little high today because I'm nervous.

Unit 6　I need to ask you some questions.

Sometimes doctors need information about their patients' personal lives, and the health of family members. Do you know your family's medical history? Are your eating and sleeping habits healthy? （時には患者本人の病歴や家族構成・病歴などについて聞くこともあります。自分の家族の病歴は知っていますか？自分のライフスタイルについて語れますか？）

KEY EXPRESSIONS

NURSES' KEY EXPRESSIONS

1. Can you please fill in this form?
   「こちらの用紙に記入をお願いします」
2. Do you smoke? How many a day?
   「タバコは吸いますか？１日にどれくらい吸いますか？」
3. Do you drink? How much and how often do you drink?
   「お酒は飲みますか？どれくらいの頻度、量を飲みますか？」
4. Have you ever had any serious illness?
   「重い病にかかった事はありますか？」
5. Do you have a family history of cancer?
   「家族でがんにかかった人はいますか？」
6. Are you currently taking any medication?
   「現在何か薬を飲んでいますか？」
7. Do you exercise regularly? How many hours a week?
   「定期的に運動はしますか？週にどれくらいしますか？」
8. Do you eat a balanced diet?
   「バランスの良い食事をとっていますか？」
9. Do you have any allergies?
   「アレルギーはありますか？」
10. Is there any chance of you being pregnant?
    「妊娠している可能性はありますか？」

PATIENTS' KEY EXPRESSIONS

1. I'm sorry. I can't read Japanese.
   「すみません。日本語が読めません」
2. I'm allergic to peanuts.
   「私にはピーナッツアレルギーがあります」

■■■ Communication Strategy ■■■
–Be an Active Listener–

One way to be active when you listen is to respond to the speaker. These words and phrases show that you are interested and that you are listening. （相手の話を聞く時は興味を示す姿勢も大切です。うなずきながら答えてみましょう。）

To show interest:	Oh really?
	Oh?
To show you are listening:	Hmmm.
	Uh-huh.
	Mm-hmm.
To show you agree:	Uh-huh.

SPEAKING PRACTICE 1

Use the key questions, coupled with the strategies to get information about your patient. （相手の会話に興味を示しながら、質問をしてみましょう。）

Patient Name _____

Tobacco: Yes / No
(____ packets / day)

Alcohol: Yes / No
(____ glasses of wine / beer / spirits
every day / ____ times a week)

Exercise: Yes / No
(____ hrs / week)

Patient Name _____

Tobacco: Yes / No
(____ packets / day)

Alcohol: Yes / No
(____ glasses of wine / beer / spirits
every day / ____ times a week)

Exercise: Yes / No
(____ hrs / week)

Unit 6   I need to ask you some questions.

MEDICAL VOCABULARY
– Illnesses and Diseases –

allergy	アレルギー	hypotension	低血圧
anemia	貧血	incontinence	失禁
appendicitis	虫垂炎	infectious disease	伝染病
asthma	ぜん息	Japanese encephalitis	日本脳炎
atopic dermatitis	アトピー性皮膚炎	leukemia	白血病
bronchitis	気管支炎	measles	はしか
cancer	癌	meningitis	髄膜炎
cataract	白内障	mental disorder**	精神障害
chickenpox	水痘	muliple sclerosis	多発性硬化症
coeliac disease	セリアック病、小児脂肪便症	mumps	おたふく風邪
		myoma of the uterus (fibroids)	子宮筋腫
common cold	風邪		
conjunctivitis	結膜炎	osteoporosis	骨粗鬆症
contact dermatitis	接触皮膚炎	otitis media	中耳炎
coronavirus	コロナウイルス	pertussis (whooping cough)	百日咳
cystitis	膀胱炎		
diabetes mellitus (DM)	糖尿病	pleurisy	胸膜炎
duodenal ulcer	十二指腸潰瘍	pneumonia	肺炎
dyspnea (shortness of breath)	呼吸困難症（息切れ）	rheumatoid arthritis	関節リウマチ
		roseola	バラ疹
eczema	湿疹	rubella (German meales)	風疹
epilepsy	癲癇（てんかん）	sleep apnea	睡眠時無呼吸
gallstone	胆石	staph infection	ブドウ球菌感染症
gastric ulcer	胃潰瘍	STD (Sexually Transmitted Disease)	性感染症
glaucoma	緑内障		
gonorrhea	淋病	streptococcosis	レンサ球菌感染症
gout	痛風	strep throat	レンサ球菌咽頭炎
heart burn	胸やけ	syphilis	梅毒
heart disease*	心臓病	tinea (athlete's foot)	水虫
hepatitis	肝炎	tonsillitis	扁桃炎
herniated disc	椎間板ヘルニア	tuberculosis (T.B.)	結核
herpes	ヘルペス	tumor	腫瘍
hives	蕁麻疹	vaginitis	膣炎
hypertension	高血圧	vertigo (dizziness)	めまい

AIDS (Acquired Immunodeficiency Syndrome) 　エイズ（後天性免疫不全症候群）

HIV (Human Immunodeficiency Virus) 　ヒト免疫不全ウイルス

* "disease"（全身または一部の構造や機能が正常を失った状態）例：lung disease, liver disease, kidney disease
** "disorder" 心身機能の不調、異常、障害や軽い病気のとき使う。例：brain disorder, intestinal disorder, genetic disorder
*** "condition"（健康の妨げになる状態や病状）例：a heart condition, a liver condition

SPEAKING PRACTICE 2

Practice the following conversation, substituting the underlined words for other time expressions and diseases.（下線の部分の言葉を入れ替えて、練習しなさい。）

N: Have you ever had any serious illness?

P: Last year, I had tuberculosis.

N: Tuberculosis?

P: Yes.

N: I see.

....

1. Three years ago....　a gastric ulcer

2. When I was nine....　whooping cough

3. Five years ago....　measles

4. Last year....　appendicitis

WORD POWER

AFFIX	MEANING	EXAMPLES
mal	悪	malignant tumor, malaise, malfunction
bene	善	benign tumor, beneficial, benefit
itis	炎症	appendicitis, dermatitis, arthritis, rhinitis
dis	非・異	disorder, disability, disease, disaster, dislocation
dia	通る	diabetes, dialysis, diaphragm, diagnosis

Unit 6　I need to ask you some questions.

WRITING PRACTICE 1

Study the affixes in the Word Power list and match the meanings with the words underlined in the sentences below. （前ページの語源のリストを見て、下記の文章の中の下線の言葉の意味を a ～ e から探しなさい。）

1. ____ Mary had a <u>malignant</u> melanoma removed.

2. ____ Tests proved the tumor to be <u>benign</u>.

3. ____ Alex was admitted to hospital with acute <u>appendicitis</u>.

4. ____ Surveys show that American postal workers tend to suffer from more stress-related mental <u>disorders</u> than other professions.

5. ____ Although Alice had to visit a <u>dialysis</u> center three times a week, she still continued to work as a nature photographer.

a. good; not harmful

b. to remove waste from blood by passing it through a machine

c. when the body does not function correctly

d. an inflamed appendix

e. bad; life-threatening

 Mini-Dictionary:

- melanoma　黒色腫
- tumor　腫瘍
- admit (to hospital)　入院する
- survey　調査

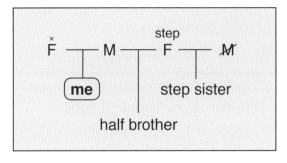

※ 右の図は、片親が離別（離婚や死亡など）し、その後再婚した場合を表しています。

※ 養子の場合

　　I'm an adopted child. I don't know my biological parents.

WRITING PRACTICE 2

Fill in the family tree chart.

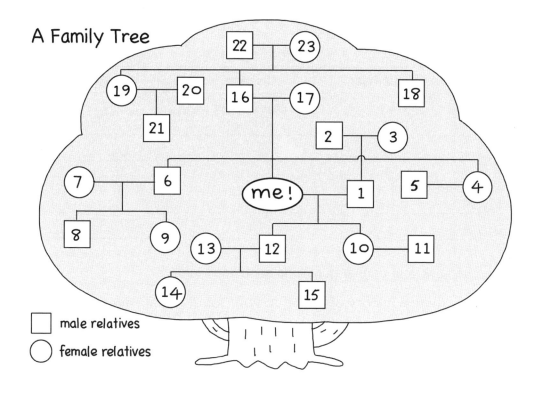

A Family Tree

□ male relatives
○ female relatives

1. _____

2. _____

3. _____

4. _____

5. _____

6. _____

7. _____

8. _____

9. _____

10. _____

11. _____

12. _____

13. _____

14. _____

15. _____

16. _____

17. _____

18. _____

19. _____

20. _____

21. _____

22. _____

23. _____

Unit 6   I need to ask you some questions.

SPEAKING PRACTICE 3

First, write an imaginary family medical history chart for yourself. Use the Illness and Diseases list to record the names of diseases. Add when they were diagnosed or for how long they had the disease. （家族の病歴を想像し、下の表を完成させましょう。）

	Family member	disease	when diagnosed
eg	*mother* *father*	*breast cancer* *diabetes*	*4 years ago* *since 2015*
1			
2			
3			
4			

Then ask your partner questions about their family.

> Is there a history of <u>cancer</u> in your family? (heart disease / diabetes)
> Is there a history of serious illness in your family?

> eg. N: Do you have a family history of serious illness? Heart disease, for example?
> P: My father has been suffering from diabetes since 2015.
> N: Are there any other family members with a history of ill health?
> P: My mother was diagnosed with breast cancer 4 years ago.

Fill in your patient's family medical history chart. （家族の病歴を聞いて、表を完成させましょう。）

Patient's Name _____

	Family member	disease	duration / diagnosed
1			
2			
3			
4			

DIALOGUE 6

First, listen to the recording. Then listen again, and fill in the blanks.

N: (1)_____ fill in this form?

P: I'm sorry. I can't read Japanese.

N: Then I'll ask you the questions. Okay? First, do you (2)_____
_____?

P: Well, I eat three meals a day, and I usually eat vegetables, meat or
fish, and rice. Good food keeps us healthy, right?

N: Uh huh. (3)_____?

P: No. I used to, but I quit four years ago.

N: Were you a heavy smoker?

P: No, only about 10 cigarettes a day.

N: Oh, I see. (4)_____?

P: Well, at restaurants or parties I'll drink a glass of wine or some
beer, but I seldom drink at home.

N: Okay. Do you sleep well, and (5)_____ do
you sleep at night?

P: I have trouble sleeping. Lately I only sleep about four or five hours.

N: Oh, really? (6) _____ regularly?

P: Yes. Since April I've been going to the gym twice a week.

N: Have you ever had (7)_____?

P: Well, I had asthma when I was a child. And about six years ago I
caught pneumonia. Last month I had bronchitis.

N: Um hmm. Do you have (8)_____ of cancer?

P: No. But my grandfather died of a heart attack at 70.

N: I see. And are you currently (9)_____ or
supplements?

P: No, not any more.

N: Are you (10)_____ any medication?

P: No. Not as far as I know.

N: Okay, that's all. Please wait here. The doctor will see you shortly.

Unit 7　Can you describe the pain?

WARM-UP

When patients enter a hospital or clinic with injuries, the nurse must ask questions about the injury and then must act quickly to help them.　Have you ever had an injury?　What questions do you think a nurse would ask a patient about an injury?（新しく入院する患者さんを迎えるときには、いろんな質問をして情報収集に努めます。ナースはどのような質問をするべきか考えましょう。）

KEY EXPRESSIONS

NURSES' KEY EXPRESSIONS

1. When did you injure yourself?
   「いつ怪我をしましたか？」
2. How did you injure your leg?
   「どのように足に怪我をしましたか？」
3. Are you in much pain?
   「痛みはどのくらいありますか？」
4. Can you describe the pain?
   「どのような痛みですか？」
5. When did you first notice the pain?
   「痛みに最初に気づいたのはいつですか？」
6. On a scale of 1-10, how would you rate your pain?
   「1 から 10 までの基準では、どれくらいの痛さがありますか？」

PATIENTS' KEY EXPRESSIONS

1. I cut my finger this morning.
   「今朝指を切りました」
2. I hurt my knee (while) playing football.
   「フットボールをしている時にひざを怪我しました」
3. It's a throbbing pain.
   「ズキズキするような痛みです」
4. It usually doesn't bother me.
   「普段は気になりません」
5. Can I have something to stop the pain?
   「痛み止めをもらう事はできますか？」

■■■ **Communication Strategy** ■■■

–Keep the conversation rolling–

To help keep the conversation moving or "rolling" along, connecting words like "so" and "and" can be used.（会話が流れるように工夫をしましょう。）

For example:

N: So ... When did you first notice the pain?

or

N: And ... Where exactly does it hurt?

or

N: Well then ... Can you tell me how you hurt yourself?

TIME VOCABULARY
– THE PAST ← NOW –

( ) ← (	) ←	yesterday	←	today
( ) ← the week before last	← (		) ←	this week
3 months ago ← (	) ←	last month	← (	)
3 years ago ← the year before last	← (		) ← (	)

WRITING PRACTICE 1

Answer the questions about yourself, or ask your partner, and record his/her answers.

1. When did you last get a flu injection?

   _____.

2. When did you last visit a farm or rural area?*

   _____.

3. When did you last do exercise or play sport?

   _____.

> **Cultural Quip**
>
> *This question is often asked in the U.K., Europe, and Australia, especially after the BSE scare in the U.K. in the early 1990's.（狂牛病発生以降、イギリスやオーストラリアでは、最近牧場や農場へ行ったかどうかをチェックされる。）

SPEAKING PRACTICE 1

Practice using the strategy, and then practice the conversation below.

P: I've <u>hurt my foot</u>.

N: And ... when did this happen?

P: <u>The day before yesterday</u>.

N: How did you injure yourself?

P: I was <u>playing tennis</u> when it happened.

N: So ... when did you first notice the pain?

P: <u>Yesterday</u>.

....

1. "... hurt my back   / last week   / lifting boxes
   / about 3 days ago"

2. "... hurt my hand   / this morning   / playing tennis
   / almost immediately"

3. "... hit my head   / yesterday   / renovating
   / last night"

4. "... hurt my leg   / the week before last / planting rice
   / last week"

5. "... cut my finger   / at lunchtime   / making lunch
   / straight away"

– Pain Scale –

On a scale of 1-10, how would you rate your pain?
（ペインスケールを用いて、患者さんに痛みの度合いを尋ねましょう。）

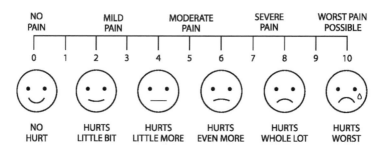

MEDICAL VOCABULARY
–Pain and Injuries–

● throbbing pain ずきずきする痛み （eg. "It's a throbbing pain."）

● stabbing pain 刺すような痛み

● splitting pain 割れるような痛み （eg. "I have a splitting headache."）

● sharp pain 激しい、鋭い痛み

● dull pain にぶい痛み

● nagging pain しつこい痛み

● numbness しびれ（感覚が無くなる）（eg. "It feels numb."）

● pins and needles しびれ（皮膚がちくちくする）（eg. "I have pins and needles."）

● sting ちくっとする痛み（虫刺されのような痛み）（eg. "It stings."）

● tingle ひりひりする痛み

● tenderness 圧痛 （eg. "It feels tender to touch."）

● fatigue / lethargy 体がだるい （eg. "I feel tired and have no energy."）

● fracture 骨折 （eg. "My arm is broken."）

● compound / open fracture 開放骨折

● simple fracture 単純骨折

● comminuted fracture 粉砕骨折

● sprain / sprained 捻挫 （eg. "I sprained my ankle."）

● swelling / swollen 腫脹 （eg. "I have swollen ankles."）

● twist / twisted 捻った （eg. "I twisted my ankle."）

● damaged ligament 傷ついた靭帯

● torn ligament 靭帯損傷 （eg. "I've pulled a muscle."）

● dislocation 脱臼 （eg. "I dislocated my shoulder"）

● acute (pain) 急性的な（痛み）

● chronic (pain) 慢性的な（痛み）

● It (The pain) comes and goes. 痛かったり、痛くなかったりする。

Cultural Quip

When recording how long the patient has had the symptoms, fractions are usually used. （症状がどのくらいの間続いているのかを分数で表します。）
eg. 3 / 7 = three days ; 6 / 52 = six weeks ; 8 / 12 = eight months

SPEAKING PRACTICE 2

Practice the conversation and expand with the examples below. Notice how shadowing keeps the conversation going. （シャドウイングのストラテジーを思い出しながら、モデルとなる会話を練習しましょう。）

N: Good morning, Mrs. Brown. How do you feel today?

P: Oh, Nurse! I had a terrible night.

N: A bad night? Why?

P: I woke up with <u>a splitting headache</u>.

N: <u>A headache</u>? Does it still hurt?

P: Yes. I couldn't sleep properly.

N: I'll bring you an analgesic for the pain. Just rest easy now.

....

1. a stabbing pain in my chest / A pain in your chest?

2. a throbbing pain in my leg / A pain in your leg?

3. nagging neck pain / Neck pain?

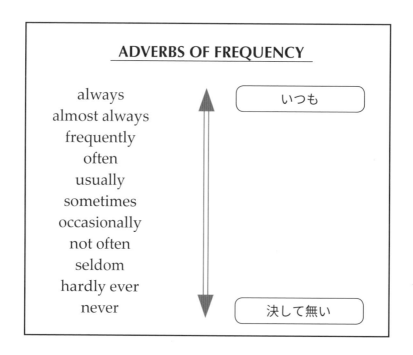

ADVERBS OF FREQUENCY

always
almost always
frequently
often
usually
sometimes
occasionally
not often
seldom
hardly ever
never

いつも

決して無い

WRITING PRACTICE 2

Ask your partner the following questions and record the answers using adverbs of frequency from the list. (頻度を表す副詞を使い、あなたのパートナーに下記の質問をして答えを記録しましょう。架空の患者さんのことでも構いません。)

When do you usually get a headache?

_____ .

Does the pain always bother you?

_____ .

Does lying down sometimes ease the pain?

_____ .

  # SPEAKING PRACTICE 3

What questions would you ask a pregnant client who has come in experiencing bleeding? (出血を訴える妊婦が病院に訪れたら、どう対応しますか？日本語のヒントを使って、会話を完成しなさい。)

P:　I'm Alison Summers. I want to see a doctor immediately.

N:　（どうしましたか？）_____

P:　I'm pregnant, and I started bleeding. I'm afraid for my baby.

N:　（母子手帳はありますか？）_____

P:　No. I left it at home, in Australia.

N:　（では、何週目ですか？）_____

P:　I'm 6 months pregnant. The 26th week, I think.

N:　（出血はいつから？）_____

P:　Last night.

N:　（出血の量は？月経と同じぐらいの量？）_____

P:　A few red spots. I hope I'm not going to lose my baby!

N:　（痛みは？陣痛？）_____

P:　No. No pain. But I often have leg cramps.

N:　（心配しないで。医師の診察はもう少しで始まります。）_____

_____

** 母子手帳 = Pregnancy Health Book / Mother-Child Health Record Book (pre & post birth)

WORD POWER

AFFIX	MEANING	EXAMPLES
a / an	欠乏・無	anaemia, anoxia, analgesic, anesthesia
frag / fract	破砕	fracture, fragile infraction, fragment
scrib / script	書く	describe, prescription, transcribe
tract	引く	traction, extract, distract, contraction
temp / chron	時	temporary, chronic, synchronize

 # WRITING PRACTICE 3

Using the information about the Greek and Latin roots above, complete the exercise.

1. ____ Sleep <u>apnea</u> is very common, and affects more than twelve million Americans.

2. ____ The ambulance brought in a boy with multiple <u>fractures</u>.

3. ____ Take this <u>prescription</u> to the nearest pharmacy, and you will get your medicine.

4. ____ The patient was in <u>traction</u> for two weeks following the accident.

5. ____ Consistent high blood pressure can cause <u>chronic</u> kidney disease.

a. broken bones
b. an order written by a doctor for a pharmacist
c. without breathing
d. for a long time; long-lasting
e. a system of weights and pulleys to straighten a broken or deformed limb

 Mini-Dictionary:

● consistent 一貫した　　　　　● kidney 腎臓

DIALOGUE 7

First, listen to the recording. Then listen again, and fill in the blanks.

Nurse: Good evening, Ms. Mason. What's the problem today?

Patient: I hurt my knee. Here.

Nurse: Are you (1)_____ ?

Patient: Yes, it's really painful.

Nurse: Can you (2)_____ ?

Patient: It's a throbbing pain.

Nurse: A throbbing pain. I see. When did you (3)_____

_____?

Patient: It started about eight weeks ago, but it comes and goes.

Nurse: Do you have (4)_____?

Patient: No, only my knee.

Nurse: (5)_____ it?

Patient: I went skiing about two months ago, and I think I hurt it then.

It (6)_____ but the day before

yesterday I ran up the stairs and (7)_____.

Nurse: Please wait here and the doctor will see you shortly.

Patient: It hurts. Can I have something (8) _____?

Nurse: I'll ask the doctor if you can be (9) _____.

... (later) We'll need some X-rays. I'm going to take you in this

wheelchair (10)_____.

Unit 8　Rest your arm on the armrest.

WARM-UP

Often a nurse must give instructions to a patient, for example to put his body into position for an X-ray or for an examination.　Think of some other possible instructions we may have to give.（看護師は患者さんが診察や検査を受けるときに様々な指示を伝えます。どのような言い方があるか、考えてみましょう。）

KEY EXPRESSIONS

NURSES' KEY EXPRESSIONS

1. Come this way.
   「こちらに来てください」
2. Sit down.
   「座ってください」
3. Roll up your sleeve.
   「袖をまくってください」

PATIENTS' KEY EXPRESSIONS

1. Where can I put my bag?
   「カバンはどこにおけばいいですか？」
2. Can I sit here?
   「ここに座ってもいいですか？」

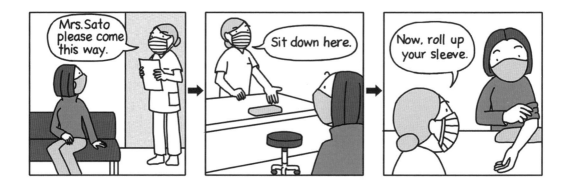

MEDICAL VOCABULARY
–Instructions–

Sit down.

Stand up.

Sit up.

Take off your shirt.

Put on this gown.

Roll up your sleeve.

Make a fist.

Relax.

Apply pressure.

Sit up on the examination table.

Breathe in.

Breathe out.

Breathe deeply.

Hold your breath.

Inhale.

Exhale.

Breathe normally.

Turn around.

Push / Don't push yet.

Lie down.

Lie on your stomach.

Lie face down.

Lie on your back.

Lie face up.

Lie on your side.

Lie on your left side.

Bend your legs.

Straighten your legs.

Fill the cup to the line.

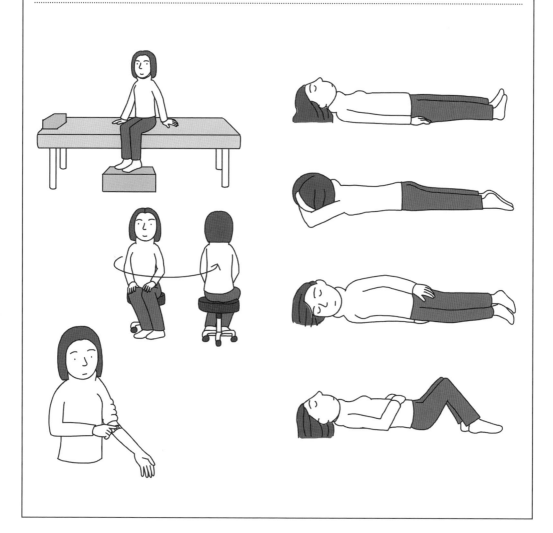

Unit 8   Rest your arm on the armrest.

SPEAKING PRACTICE 1

Practice the following conversations with a friend. Do the actions as well as the speaking. （下の表現を実際に動作をしながら練習しましょう。）

②⑥ Taking a blood sample:（採血）

N: Sit down here please.
　　Roll up your sleeve.
　　Put your arm on the armrest.
　　Make a fist.
　　.................
　　Now relax.
　　Apply pressure on this point.

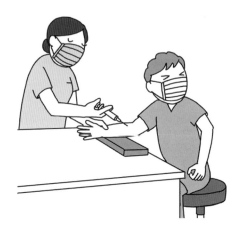

②⑦ Taking blood pressure:（血圧を図る）

N: Sit down here please.
　　Take off your coat.
　　Put your arm on the armrest.
　　Relax.

②⑧ Giving an intramuscular injection:（筋肉注射をする）

N: I'm going to give you an injection into the muscle here at the top of your arm.
　　It might hurt a little.
　　I'll count to three. 1… 2… (inject).. 3. Well done.

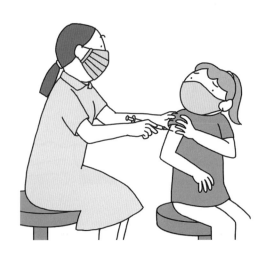

To relax the patient when you must take a blood sample or give an injection, you can *give her/him a compliment*. A compliment is saying something nice about someone. (患者さんをリラックスさせるためには、患者さんの身近なことについてほめてあげることも大切です。)

For example,

　　Nice glasses.

　　　or

　　I like your red sweater.

SPEAKING PRACTICE 2

Compliment the person, or people near you.

Hair:	Your hair looks lovely like that! Who do you get to cut it?
Clothing:	That color really suits you!
	That's a lovely dress you're wearing, Mrs. Green.
	That's an interesting tie you're wearing Mr. Williams.
Accessories:	What a beautiful ring! Did you buy that in Japan?
	That's a nice hat. You're wise to wear a hat in this weather.
	They're unusual glasses. Are they new?
Family:	I hear your son got into University. Congratulations!
	I hear you're a grandmother now. That's wonderful!

WRITING PRACTICE 1

Fill in the blanks to complete this exercise which includes giving instructions. (尿検査・血液検査の場合) Choose words from the selection below.

1. For a urinalysis the nurse needs a (　　　　　　　　) sample.
2. First (　　　　　　) a little into the toilet; then (　　　　　) a midstream specimen in the cup provided.
3. (　　　　　　) the cup to about one-third.
4. For a blood sample the nurse must (　　　　　　　) blood.
5. (　　　　　　) this cotton to your arm until it stops bleeding.
6. Don't (　　　　　　) or massage it.

　　(collect / urinate / rub / draw / urine / fill / press)

WORD POWER

AFFIX	MEANING	EXAMPLES
spec / spect	みる	inspect, specimen, retrospect, speculate
pan	全	pandemic, panacea, panotitis, pancreas
tort	ねじる	tort, tourniquet, distortion, contort
ante	前	antenatal, anterior, antemortem, antepartum
post	後	postnatal, posterior, postmortem, postpartum

WRITING PRACTICE 2

Using the information about the Greek and Latin roots above, complete the exercise.

1. ____ The <u>postmortem</u> examination showed that the woman had been poisoned.

2. ____ Her face <u>contorted</u> with pain during the procedures.

3. ____ In <u>retrospect</u>, Ronda's unusual fatigue was a warning sign predicting her heart attack.

4. ____ Many medical doctors consider Vitamin C the <u>panacea</u> for all diseases.

5. ____ Before the birth of her first child, Mrs. Jones visited the <u>antenatal</u> care clinic regularly.

....

a. before birth
b. looking back
c. after death
d. twist violently
e. a cure all

Mini-Dictionary:
- poison　毒を与える
- procedures　処置
- fatigue　疲労
- predict　予言する・予測する
- Vitamin C　ビタミンC

DIALOGUE 8

First, listen to the recording. Then listen again, and fill in the blanks.

● *In Pathology:*

N: We need to do (1)_____ and a blood test. First, let's get (2)_____.

P: Okay. What should I do?

N: (3)_____ to the toilet down the hall on the right. First urinate a little into the toilet. Then urinate into the cup.

P: How much into the cup?

N: Fill the cup about (4)_____.

P: What should I do with it?

N: (5)_____ the special window beside the hand basin.

● *A few minutes later*

P: Um... Excuse me. What other tests do I need to take?

N: Well, now we need (6)_____.

P: How much blood will you draw?

N: About 20 cc. Please sit down. You can put your bag in the basket. Okay. First, take off your sweater. Oh, I like your red sweater.

P: Thank you. My daughter made it for me.

N: Oh? How nice! Now, (7)_____ and hold out your arm.

P: Like this?

N: Yes, that's good. Now (8)_____, like this, and squeeze your hand.

P: I don't like needles.

N: You'll feel just a little pinch. That's good. (9)_____ now.

P: It didn't hurt at all.

N: Press this cotton to your arm and (10)_____ for a few minutes till the blood stops.

Unit 8   Rest your arm on the armrest.

Unit 9　Please make a follow-up appointment.

A nurse always wears a watch and often records the time of treatment or medication, etc. In a clinic, a nurse often makes appointments for patients. Telling time and understanding days of the week and months are important. （病院では患者さんに正確な時間を知ることや伝えることが大切です。薬を飲む時間や次回の診察の日付などを正しく伝えましょう。）

KEY EXPRESSIONS

NURSES' KEY EXPRESSIONS

1. Can you come in next week Thursday?
　「次の木曜日に来ることはできますか？」
2. How about Friday?
　「金曜日はどうでしょうか？」
3. Is 3 p.m. convenient?/ Is 3 o'clock in the afternoon okay?
　「午後3時のご都合は？」
4. When do you expect to come in next?
　「次回はいつ来られますか？」
5. We'll see you in 6 weeks time then.
　「では、6週間後にお越しください」

PATIENTS' KEY EXPRESSIONS

1. I need to make an appointment to see the doctor.
　「診察の予約をお願いします」
2. That's not a good day for me.
　「その日は都合が良くないです」
3. I can come in the week after next.
　「再来週に来ることはできます」

■■■ Communication Strategy ■■■
–Paraphrasing–

There are times when you may have to *paraphrase* and repeat what you have just said. For example, children may not know certain medical terms, or people who have learnt English as their third or fourth foreign language may also have difficulty. （時にはある表現を別の表現で言い換えることも必要です。例えば、子供や英語を母国語としない人たちは、難しい医学用語を理解できないことがあります。）

Eg. a flu shot   →   an injection for influenza

Any other symptoms?   →   Do you have any other problems or pain?

a stomachache   →   a tummy ache（幼児語）

MEDICAL VOCABULARY
–TELLING THE TIME–

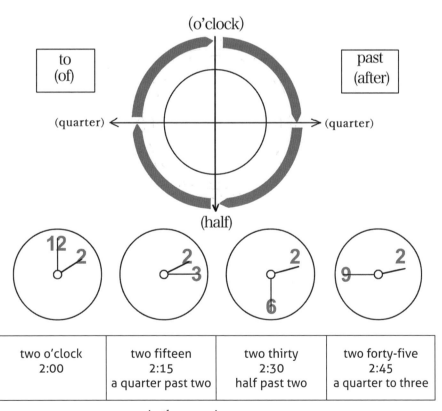

two o'clock 2:00	two fifteen 2:15 a quarter past two	two thirty 2:30 half past two	two forty-five 2:45 a quarter to three

a.m. = in the morning
p.m. = in the afternoon = in the evening = at night

WRITING PRACTICE 1

Complete the chart.

| six fifteen | = | 6:15 | = | a quarter past six |

nine fifty	=	9:50	=	(1)_____
three oh five	=	(2)_____	=	five past three
(3)_____	=	4:15	=	a quarter past four
two forty-five	=	2:45	=	(4)_____
eight twenty	=	8:20	=	(5)_____
(6)_____	=	7:30	=	half past seven

Now complete the clock faces:

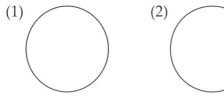

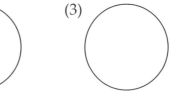

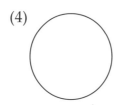

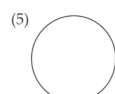

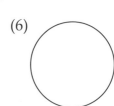

Cultural Quip

Nurses will sometimes use a 24-hour clock when talking about their shifts. However, with the patient, they will use ordinary time expressions. (看護師同士は24時間時計を使うことがありますが、患者さんとは通常の時間の言いまわしを使うように気を付けましょう。)

For example: 16:00 = "sixteen hundred hours" amongst nurses
but 16:00 = "four o'clock in the afternoon" with patients

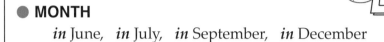

MEDICAL VOCABULARY
– Time –

- **YEAR**
  in 1957, *in* 2003, *in* 2020

- **MONTH**
  in June, *in* July, *in* September, *in* December

- **DAY**
  on Monday, *on* Tuesday, *on* Wednesday, *on* Sunday

- **DATE**
  on the 1st (fir**st**), *on* the 3rd (thi**rd**), *on* the 16th (sixteen**th**),
  on the 22nd (twenty-seco**nd**), *on* the 30th (thirtie**th**)

- **TIME**
  at three o'clock, *at* midnight, *at* twelve noon, *at* 4:15

WRITING PRACTICE 2

Answer the following questions about time and dates. Look at a calendar when necessary. （必要に応じてカレンダーを見て以下の質問に答えて下さい。）

1. What time do you get up in the morning?

   _____.

2. What time does this English class finish?

   _____.

3. The appointment is for Monday, next week. What date is that?

   _____.

4. The patient has an appointment with Dr. Suzuki at 11 o'clock on the last Friday of next month. What date is that?

   _____.

5. Mariko will be admitted on the 16th. What day is that?

   _____.

TIME VOCABULARY
– Now → The Future –

today   → (   ) → (   ) → (   )

(   ) →   **next week**   → (   ) → (   )

(   ) → (   ) → (   ) →   **in 3 months time**

(   ) → (   ) →   **the year after next**   → (   )

Cultural Qulp

[来週の水曜日] English speakers might say "a week from Wednesday" while other might say "Wednesday week." All English speakers understand both expressions.

SPEAKING PRACTICE 1

Ask your partner questions about the future. Record their answers. Use your imagination. (未来のことを尋ねてみましょう。想像したことでもかまいませんので、質問をし相手の答えを記録しましょう。)

● Amongst friends:

1. When do you expect to graduate?

   _____.

2. When do you expect to have your next hospital prac?

   _____.

3. When do you expect to leave for overseas?

   _____.

● With your patient:

4. When do you expect to see the doctor next?

   _____.

5. When do you expect to have the operation?

   _____.

SPEAKING PRACTICE 2

Practice the dialogue about making an appointment with a partner, and continue with the substitutions. （診察予約をする時の会話を練習しましょう。）

N: When can you come in for your (A)flu shot?

P: How about (B)next Thursday?

N: Thursday is fine. How about (C)2 o'clock (in the afternoon)?

P: That's fine.

N: Good. We'll see you next Thursday at 2:00 then.

....

1. (A)tests   / (B)the day after tomorrow / (C)4:30
                                                                  (in the afternoon)

2. next blood test   / next month on the 11th / 11:00
                                                                 (in the morning)

3. next appointment / next week on Friday   / 9:30
                                                                 (in the morning)

WORD POWER

AFFIX	MEANING	EXAMPLES
ject	投げる	subject, reject, injection, autoinjector
ann / enn	年	annual, biennial, anniversary, biannual
gen	生きる	generation, genes, gender, pathogen
fin	制限・終り	final, infinite, confine, definite
multi / poly	多数の	multiple, polydactylism, multilingual, polymyositis, polyphagia

WRITING PRACTICE 3

Using the information about the Greek and Latin roots above, complete the exercise.

1. ____ The patient was put into <u>confinement</u> after he was diagnosed with SARS.

2. ____ <u>Polyphagia</u> is frequently a result of abnormal blood glucose levels.

3. ____ The <u>annual</u> cost for National Health Insurance where I live is 40,000 yen.

4. ____ At the Mercy Children's Hospital, staff provide care for patients with <u>genetic</u> mental disorders.

5. ____ One well-known treatment for blue spider veins is by <u>injecting</u> a solution into them.

....

    a. eating a lot, excessive eating

    b. limiting the movement

    c. force a fluid into the body; give medicine by use of a needle

    d. original; (illnesses) that are carried from father to son and on to grandson

    e. yearly

Mini-Dictionary:

- glucose　ブドウ糖
- solution　液体
- spider veins　クモ状血管道腫
- provide　与える

DIALOGUE 9

First, listen to the recording. Then listen again, and fill in the blanks.

Nurse: Good morning. Nishimura Clinic. May I help you?

Patient: Yes, my name is Denise Winner, and I need (1)_____ _____ the doctor, please.

Nurse: What's the trouble?

Patient: No trouble. I just need a flu shot.

Nurse: (2)_____? Could you please repeat that?

Patient: I want to get a flu shot... (3)_____ against influenza.

Nurse: I see. If you have your registration card, could you please tell me the registration number?

Patient: Yes. My registration number is 7098-02.

Nurse: 7098-02. Thank you. Could you come in (4)_____

          _____; Thursday, the 16th ?

Patient: That's (5)_____ for me. I work on Thursdays. How about Friday, the 17th ?

Nurse: I'm sorry. The doctor isn't (6)_____. How about next week Monday, the 20th ?

Patient: That would be fine. What time?

Nurse: Is 3 p.m. (7) _____?

Patient: Pardon?

Nurse: Is 3 o'clock (8)_____ a suitable time for you?

Patient: Yes. Three is fine.

Nurse: Good. Then your appointment is set for 3 p.m. next Monday, November 20th.

Patient: Thank you.

Nurse: And what is your (9)_____, Ms. Winner?

Patient: Do you mean my number at work?

Nurse: Yes, the number that you (10)_____ during the daytime.

Patient: It's 082-920-7436.

Nurse: 082-920-7436. Ok, we'll see you next Monday at 3 o'clock then. Good-bye.

Patient: Thank you. Good-bye.

Unit 10 Take this medicine after meals.

WARM-UP

Japanese have a habit of keeping a medicine chest that is filled regularly by traveling salesmen. Westerners often prepare their own chests including items they use most often. What do you have in your medicine chest?
（日本には常備薬という薬屋さんがしばしば薬を補充しに来る習慣がありますが、欧米ではよく使うものを引き出しの中に備えていることが多いです。あなたの家の救急箱にはどんな薬が入ってますか？）

KEY EXPRESSIONS

NURSES' KEY EXPRESSIONS

1. Here is your medicine.
   「こちらがお薬になります」
2. Take this medicine after meals.
   「これを食後に服用してください」
3. Use this cream when you feel itchy.
   「かゆみのある時はこのクリームを使ってください」
4. Take one tablet three times a day.
   「1日3回この錠剤を1錠服用して下さい」
5. Use one or two drops per eye.
   「1・2滴それぞれの目にさしてください」

PATIENTS' KEY EXPRESSIONS

1. How often should I take these tablets?
   「どのくらいの頻度でこの錠剤を服用すればいいですか？」
2. I have difficulty swallowing big tablets.
   「大きい錠剤を服用するのは難しいです」
3. Can I crush the tablets?
   「錠剤を粉末にする事はできますか？」

MEDICAL VOCABULARY
– Medicine –

● MEDICINE FOR INTERNAL USE ［内服薬］

tablet	錠剤	
pill	錠剤	（The Pill = contraceptive = 避妊の薬）

　　※ Older people tend to prefer the use of "pill" over "tablet".

capsule	カプセル
syrup	シロップ
powdered medicine	粉薬（漢方薬）
granular medicine	顆粒状の薬

● MEDICINE FOR EXTERNAL USE ［外用薬］

cream	軟膏・クリーム（白っぽい粘稠性の薬）
ointment	軟膏（油性膏薬）
powder	パウダー
spray	スプレー
suppository	座薬
gargle	うがいの薬
eye drops	眼薬・点眼薬（nose drops = 点鼻薬、ear drops = 耳点滴薬）
compress	湿布（hot pack = 温パック、ice pack = 氷パック）

● GENERAL TYPES OF MEDICINE

antibiotics	抗生剤
antiseptic	消毒剤
antipyretic	解熱剤
analgesic	鎮痛剤・痛み止め（pain killer）
cough medicine	風邪薬
throat lozenges	のど飴（トローチ）
laxatives	下剤
binding medicine	下痢止め（medicine for diarrhea）
sleeping pills	睡眠薬

■■■ Communication Strategy ■■■
–Check for understanding–

You can check to make sure that your patient understands your advice or instructions, by asking some simple questions.（患者さんが自分の指示を理解しているかどうか、時々確認しましょう。）

For example:

Okay?	Do you follow me?
Alright?	Do you understand?

SPEAKING PRACTICE

Practice the following conversation with your partner, substituting words from the aches, pains or diseases lists and from the kinds of medicine list.

P: I have <u>a sore throat</u>. What do you recommend?

N: The doctor says you should <u>take these throat lozenges</u>. Okay?

P: Alright.

....

1. sore eyes / use these eye drops
2. a stomachache / take this powdered medicine
3. an itchy foot / use this cream when it is itchy
4. diarrhea / take this binding medicine
5. a sore calf / use this spray to ease the muscle pain

INSTRUCTIONS FOR TAKING MEDICINES

HOW	HOW MUCH	WHAT	HOW OFTEN	WHEN
Take	1	tablet	once a day	before going to bed.
Take	2	capsules	twice a day	morning and night.
Take	1	sachet	three times a day	after meals.
Use	2~3	drops	every four hours.	
Use		this cream		when you feel pain.

* Some countries measure liquid medicine by teaspoons per dose or mls per dose. （国によっては、服用量を「1メモリ」とは言わず「小さじ1杯」又は「5ミリ」と指示する。）
    Eg. 5 mls per dose. (5mls = 1tsp)
* British or Australian speakers might say sachets while Americans say envelopes.
* 日本語では錠剤もカプセルも「1錠、2錠…」と数えますが、英語だと1 capsule, 2 tablets 等と、形や容器に合わせて数えます。

WRITING PRACTICE 1

Write out the following instructions for your patient.

1) このカプセル1錠を毎朝食後に飲んでください。（take）

   _____.

2) この目薬を2・3滴、一日4回点眼してしてください。（use）

   _____.

3) このシロップを5ミリ（1メモリ）、一日二回飲んでください。（take）

   _____.

4) このスプレーを（筋肉が）痛いときに使ってください。（use）

   _____.

5) この鎮痛剤を、頭痛がひどいときに2錠飲んでください。（take）

   _____.

WRITING PRACTICE 2

Look at the medicine cabinet below, and explain what is in it.

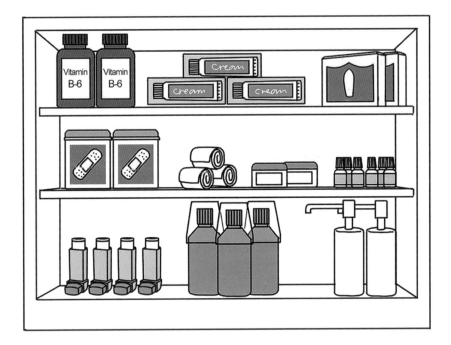

1. Where is the inhaler?

   _____.

2. Where is the ointment?

   _____.

3. Where are the suppositories?

   _____.

4. What other medicines are on the top shelf?

   _____.

5. What other medicines are on the middle shelf?

   _____.

6. What other medicines are on the bottom shelf?

   _____.

WORD POWER

AFFIX	MEANING	EXAMPLES
flu / flux	流れ・滑らか	influenza, fluid, fluctuate, reflux
ceive / cept	取る・受ける	contraceptive, conceive, receive
anti	対立	antibiotics, antiseptic, antibacterial.
ply / plex	折り重ねる	multiply, complex, reply, solar plexus
sed / sid	座る・静か	sedative, subside, sedentary, sediment

 # WRITING PRACTICE 3

Study the affixes in the Word Power list and match the meanings with the words underlined in the sentences below. （上記の語源のリストを見て、下記の文章の中の下線の言葉の意味を a ～ e から探しなさい。）

1. ____ Researchers are trying to develop an <u>antivenin</u> for the Australian box jellyfish.

2. ____ In one survey, it was found that, of patients aged 70 or over, more females than males presented with <u>multiple</u> fractures.

3. ____ In aromatherapy, allspice and cloves are considered to be natural <u>sedatives</u>.

4. ____ To keep from getting dehydrated during the hot months, be sure to drink plenty of <u>fluids</u>.

5. ____ Can <u>contraceptives</u> be bought over the counter in Japan?

a. watery matter

b. a medicine to counter the effects of poison from insects or land and sea creatures

c. a drug that stops women from getting pregnant

d. in many places; having many parts

e. (a drug) to calm people

 Mini-Dictionary:
- jellyfish　くらげ
- present (v)　（症状を）呈する、（病の兆候が）みられる
- aromatherapy　アロマセラピー
- buy over the counter　（処方箋なしで）カウンターで買う
- dehydrated　脱水
- natural　自然

DIALOGUE 10

First, listen to the recording. Then listen again, and fill in the blanks.

Nurse: Your medicine is ready, Jean.

Jean: What kind of medicine is it?

Nurse: This is your cold medicine. This bottle contains cough syrup.

Jean: How often should I take it?

Nurse: Take one measure (1)_____.

Jean: To the line. Okay. And what's in this packet?

Nurse: This packet contains some more cold medicine. Take one white tablet (2)_____, before meals.

Jean: I have difficulty swallowing big tablets. Can I crush it?

Nurse: Yes, but be sure to (3)_____ a full glass of water. Do you understand?

Jean: Uh-huh. (4)_____, with water. How long should I take them for?

Nurse: Take them for 5 days.

Jean: For 5 days. Okay.

Nurse: This packet has some red capsules in it. They are (5)_____. Take them twice a day when necessary, but keep (6)_____ between each dose.

Jean: Twice a day if I get feverish? All right. And what's this?

Nurse: These sachets contain blue (7)_____ for your stomach.

Jean: But I don't have a stomachache.

Nurse: Well, sometimes cold medicine can (8)_____.

Jean: Should I also take these with a glass of water?

Nurse: Yes. But (9)_____ while you are taking these medicines.

Jean: Not even an occasional glass of wine?

Nurse: This medication includes antibiotics. Alcohol may cause a bad reaction. (10)_____?

Jean: All right. If I need more cough medicine, can I come back to get more?

Nurse: Yes, of course. Please come again if the symptoms don't improve. Take care!

Unit 11　Your operation will be this afternoon.

WARM-UP

Foreign patients who need to have surgery in Japan are often very worried about what will happen to them. One reason for this is the language barrier, the other is lack of knowledge about the procedures. Do you know anyone who has gone through an operation?（外国籍の患者さんが日本で手術を受ける際、言葉の壁によって非常に不安になります。あなたの周りで手術を経験のある人はいますか？手術について、心配なことはありましたか？）

KEY EXPRESSIONS

> ### NURSES' KEY EXPRESSIONS
>
> 1. Your operation is scheduled at 3 this afternoon.
>   「手術は午後3時に予定しています」
> 2. Your doctor is very experienced.
>   「主治医は経験が豊富です」
> 3. Did you bring the signed consent form?
>   「署名した同意書は持ってきましたか？」
> 4. Don't eat or drink anything after 9 o'clock.
>   「9時以降は飲食しないでください」
> 5. I'm going to take you to the operating theatre.
>   「手術室にご案内します」

> ### PATIENTS' KEY EXPRESSIONS
>
> 1. I'm worried about the surgery.
>   「手術のことが心配です」
> 2. How long will I be under (anesthetic)?
>   「どのくらい麻酔状態は続きますか？」

■■■ **Communication Strategy** ■■■

–Longer equals politer–

Simple sentences are easier to say, and quicker to share information. However, longer sentences sound *more polite*, and have the added advantage of *relaxing the patient* because they sound softer. Where appropriate, try to use longer sentences. (短い方が言いやすいかもしれませんが、長く滑らかに言った方が丁寧でソフトに聞こえます。)

I will ～　　　　　　よりも　I'm going to ～

Change clothes here.　よりも　You can change in here. Take your clothes off and put on the surgical gown that has been provided.

WRITING PRACTICE 1

Practice the following sentences, using "I'm going to ～ ." to lengthen the sentences and inform the patient of what you are about to do.

1) これからおなかの毛を剃ります。

　　_____.

2) これからオペ室に案内します。(operating theatre / operating room)

　　_____.

3) これからカテーテルを外します。(catheter)

　　_____.

4) これから食事を持ってきます。

　　_____.

5) これから点滴を開始します。(I.V. drip)

　　_____.

6) 明日の朝、手術前に、浣腸をします。(enema)

　　_____.

MEDICAL VOCABULARY
– Operations –

● SURGERY [外科手術]

angioplasty	血管形成	hysterectomy	子宮摘出
appendectomy	虫垂切除	laser surgery	レーザー手術
brain surgery	脳外科手術	laparotomy	腹腔切開
biopsy	生検	lumpectomy	腫瘍摘出
cataract surgery	白内障手術	mastectomy	乳房切除
caesarean section	帝王切開	open heart surgery	開心術
coronary artery bypass	冠状動脈バイパス	pneumonectomy	肺切除
cosmetic surgery	美容外科手術	prostatectomy	前立腺切除
craniotomy	開頭術	tonsillectomy	扁桃摘出
gastrectomy	胃切除	varicotomy	静脈瘤切開
hemorrhoidectomy	痔核切除	vasectomy	精管切除

● ANESTHESIA [麻酔]

general anesthetic	全身麻酔	epidural anesthetic	硬膜外麻酔
local anesthetic	局所麻酔	spinal anesthetic	脊椎麻酔

WORD POWER

AFFIX	MEANING	EXAMPLES
ectomy / tomy	除去・切開	appendectomy, tonsillectomy, myomectomy
tact / tang	触覚	tactile, tangible, contact, contagious
cid / cis	切る・殺す	incision, scissors, suicide, concise
spir	息	respiration, perspire, expire, inspire, aspire
hemo	血	hemorrhage, hemorrhoids, hematoma

WRITING PRACTICE 2

Using the information about the Greek and Latin roots above, complete the exercise.

1. ____ After the accident, he was put on an artificial <u>respirator</u>.

2. ____ <u>Contact</u> transmission is the most prevalent way contagious infections can spread to medical workers.

3. ____ Naomi was rushed to hospital with a subarachnoid <u>hemorrhage</u>.

4. ____ Mrs. Bryant is expected to be admitted for a <u>lumpectomy</u> next Wednesday.

5. ____ Some <u>insecticides</u> can also be extremely harmful to humans.

....

   a. a substance that kills insects

   b. to touch (something); to get in touch with (someone)

   c. to cut and remove a lump (usually in the breast)

   d. bleeding from a ruptured blood vessel

   e. (man-made) breathing system

Mini-Dictionary:

● artificial 人工の   ● harmful 有害
● arachnoid くも膜

SPEAKING PRACTICE 1

Practice the following dialogue and continue with the substitutions.（以下の会話例を練習し、下線部の語句を入れ替えて言ってみましょう。）

P: Nurse, what time will my operation be?

N: Your <u>appendectomy</u> is scheduled at <u>3 this afternoon</u>. Don't eat or drink anything <u>from now on</u>.

....

1. caesarean section / 10 tomorrow morning / after 9 o'clock tonight

2. hysterectomy   / 2 this afternoon   / from now on

3. varicotomy   / 1 tomorrow afternoon / after midnight tonight

4. lumpectomy   / 9 tomorrow morning / after 6 o'clock tonight

SPEAKING PRACTICE 2

Patient Observations 患者さんを観察する

When doing your morning rounds, you will need to ask the patient about any physical changes, and you will need to check the patient's vital signs. Ask your classmate the regular morning observation questions.（朝の観察のとき、必ず生命微候（脈拍、血圧、など）の現状を調べます。場合によってはT・P・B.P.・In（摂取）・Out（排泄）だけで良いかもしれませんが、呼吸・感触などを調べる必要がある場合もあります。）

* 全体 <u>General Condition</u>:   How are you feeling today?

                                    Did you sleep well?

                                    I'm going to do my routine observation check.

* 体温 <u>Temperature</u>:   What was your temperature this morning?

                                    患者さんがまだ調べてなければ

                                    I'm going to take your temperature.

> ### *Cultural Quip*
>
> In western countries, patients rarely take their own temperature. Previously, a patient's oral temperature was usually taken, however, nowadays an ear thermometer is used. During the morning rounds, many nurses now take a portable vital signs monitor with them.（西洋では、入院中自分で自分の体温を測ることは殆どない。舌の下・耳の中に看護師が体温計を置き、測ることになる。）

* 呼吸 <u>Respiration</u>:   I'm going to listen to your chest.

* 脈拍 <u>Pulse</u>:   I'm going to check your pulse.

* 血圧 <u>Blood Pressure</u>:   I'm going to take your blood pressure.

* 食欲 <u>Appetite</u>:   How much of your meals did you eat yesterday?（答えには、「何割」よりも 3/4 などの 4 等分を使用する。almost all（ほとんど：9 割）almost nothing（ほとんどない：1 割）も使える。

* 排尿 <u>Urine</u>:   How many times did you urinate yesterday?

* 排便 <u>Bowel movement</u>:   Did you have a bowel movement yesterday?

> ### *Cultural Quip*
>
> In England, nurses will sometimes ask "How many times did you pass water?" Young children may not know the words "urinate" or "bowel". You may need to say: "How many times did you wee / pee? / "Do number 1?" and: "Do a poo / poop?" / "do number 2?"（難しい表現がわからない場合もあるので、子どもに対しては、子どもがよく使う言葉を使った方がよいでしょう。）

SPEAKING PRACTICE 3

クラスメートに朝の観察の質問を聞き、生命徴候をチェックしてください。
Morning rounds: Review the notes for Mr. Sellers.

O/E （診察）（外見＋体温）
　　　on examination (General Condition)
ENT　（耳鼻咽喉）Ears, Nose and Throat
RS　　（呼吸器系）Respiratory System
CVS　（循環器系）Cardio-vascular System (P+BP)
GIS　　（消化器系）Gastro-intestinal System （摂取）
GUS　（泌尿生殖器系）Genito-urinary System（排泄）
CNS　（中枢神経系）Central Nervous System

c/o　　complaining of
T　　　Temperature
P　　　Pulse
BP　　Blood Pressure
HS　　Heart Sounds
BM　　Bowel Movement （L2 = Large Type 2）
b.r.p. bathroom privileges = 自由にトイレへ
voided = urinated

Patient Name	_Joseph SELLERS_
O/E:	T 37.4°C
	ambulant
	showered unassisted
	"didn't sleep well"
ENT:	c/o sore throat
RS:	chest clear SpO2 98
CVS:	P 75 bpm. BP 120/75
	HS normal
GIS:	good appetite,
	ate 80% of meal
	BM L2
GUS:	b.r.p.
	voided ×6
CNS:	

Check the obsevations for Joseph Sellers. Then use the expressions to glean the information for Mr. Pile and Ms. Scott. （セラーズ氏の朝の観察の記録を見本とし、自分の患者さんの記録を書き込みなさい。）

Patient Name _____
O/E
CVS
GIS
GUS

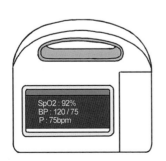

SpO2 : 92%
BP : 120/75
P : 75bpm

A（ナース）→ B（患者）
患者情報：名前：Ernie Pile
熱が39C あり、咳がすると言う。
脈は 96 b.p.m.。血圧は 150/92。
食事は半分くらいしか食べていない。
排尿は7回、排便は1回。

A（患者）← B（ナース）
患者情報：名前：Jennifer Scott
微熱があり 37.1C、身体がだるいと言う。
脈は 62 b.p.m.。血圧は 92/60。
食事は3分の1くらいしか食べていない。
排尿は4回、排便はゼロ。

WRITING PRACTICE 3

Interview your patient and write out a short report about them. Use the Sellers example.（患者に朝の問診をし、レポートに記録して下さい。）

Daily Progress Report

Patient Name   _Joseph SELLERS_   Date   _22nd May 2020_

Vital signs: temperature 37.4℃, blood pressure 120/75, pulse 75 b.p.m, oxygen level 98.
Chest is clear. Patient says he didn't sleep well, and complains of sore throat.
Patient is ambulant and showered unassisted. Patient ate 80% of dinner.

Daily Progress Report

Patient Name   _____   Date   _____

_____
_____
_____

DIALOGUE 11

First, listen to the recording. Then listen again, and fill in the blanks.

Nurse: Good morning, Mrs. Baker.

Mrs. B: Good morning, nurse. Well, today's the day, huh?

Nurse: (1)_____ about your surgery?

Mrs. B: Yes. Very!

Nurse: Well, let me explain a little about what is going to happen.
Perhaps that will (2)_____.

Mrs. B: Oh, please do!

Nurse: First, you'll need to take a shower and wash your hair (3)_____
_____ I'll give you.

Mrs. B: Yes, I know about that. That's to reduce (4)_____
_____, right?

Nurse: Yes. Then I'm going to shave your abdomen.

Mrs. B: Oh?

Nurse: Yes. Then I'm going to start your IV drip and (5)_____
_____.

Mrs. B: Will that be when I'm already in theatre?

Nurse: You'll feel drowsy along the way. But you'll be (6)_____
_____ for the operation.

Mrs. B: How long will I be under?

Nurse: Oh, for about two hours I guess.

Mrs. B: And what will happen afterwards? Will I come back to this
room straight away?

Nurse: If there are no complications I think you will be brought here.

Mrs. B: If there are no complications? What?

Nurse: Oh, please don't worry. Doctor Tanaka is (7)_____
_____ with hysterectomies.

Mrs. B: What about after I come back?

Nurse: When you wake you may (8)_____.
You'll also feel a little sore for a while.

Mrs. B: When can I get up and eat ordinarily.

Nurse: Tonight you'll be given (9)_____,
and as soon as bowel functions return you'll be on an
ordinary diet.

Mrs. B: Oh? That doesn't sound so bad then. And when will the
stitches come out?

Nurse: After about a week. Don't worry. You'll be fine, Mrs. Baker.
Now, did you bring (10)_____?

Mrs. B: Yes. Here it is.

Nurse: Thank you.

Unit 12 Are you feeling more comfortable now?

WARM-UP

Patient comfort is important in any situation. A speedy recovery is related to a decrease in stress and an improvement in comfort. What can nurses do to improve the comfort of their patients?（患者さんの痛みを和らげるために、看護師はどんな工夫をすればいいでしょうか？）

KEY EXPRESSIONS

NURSES' KEY EXPRESSIONS

1. Are you feeling more comfortable now, Mr. Collins?
   「コリンズさん、ご気分はだいぶ良くなられましたか？」
2. Do you have any dietary restrictions?
   「何か食事制限をしていますか？」
3. I'm going to change your sheets for you.
   「シーツを変えたいと思います」
4. Would you like me to open the curtains for you?
   「カーテンを開けたほうがよろしいですか？」

PATIENTS' KEY EXPRESSIONS

1. I'm a vegetarian.
   「私はベジタリアンです」
2. I can't have a blood transfusion.
   「私は輸血ができません」
3. I want to see a priest.
   「司祭に会いたいです」
4. Nurse, I feel hot.
   「看護師さん、暑いです」

● Emotional Care and Personal Comfort
（イタリック体の部分は患者さんの使用する表現です）

◆ DIETARY
Do you have any dietary restrictions?
> *I'm (a) vegetarian. / I'm (a) vegan. / I don't eat meat or fish.*
> *I'm a diabetic.*
> *I'm (a) coeliac.*
> *I can't eat foods containing gluten.*
> *I'm allergic to milk products. / I can't eat cheese.*
> *I'm lactose intolerant.*

Common food allergies:
> *milk, eggs, nuts, shellfish, fish, soy, wheat, buckwheat*

◆ RELIGIOUS
Do you have any restrictions or requirements because of your religion?
> *I can't have a blood transfusion.* (Jehovah's Witness)
> *I can't have pork.* (Islamic)
> *Do you serve Halal food?* (Islamic)
> *I can't have any beef.* (Hindu)
> *I can only eat kosher food.* (food prepared under Jewish regulations)
> *I want to see a priest.* (Catholic - in cases where the patient may die soon)

◆ HYGIENE (BODY and ORAL)
> Here are some towels for you to wipe down your body.
> Would you like me to wipe you down?
> Have your brushed your teeth yet?
> Would you like me to help you brush your teeth?
> Here are some clean pajamas for you.
> I'm going to change your sheets now.

◆ PERSONAL COMFORT
> Are you comfortable?
> Are you cold? / Are you hot?
> Would you like me to move your pillow higher?
> Would you like me to bring you another blanket?
> Would you like me to raise the backrest?
> Would you like me to raise the knee rest?

◆ STRESS
> Are you worried about your illness?
> Can your family come today?
> Visiting hours are from 2 to 4 in the afternoon.

SPEAKING PRACTICE 1

Practice the sample conversations with a partner, and then expand using the hints for other questions or expressions from each section. （以下に例として あげた２つの会話を練習し、下のヒントを参考にして会話を続けましょう。）

● **Asking for information**

N: Do you have any <u>dietary restrictions</u>, Ms. Collins?

P: Yes. <u>I'm allergic to shellfish.</u> I can't eat oysters or prawns.

....

N		P
1. dietary restrictions?	→	allergic to nuts (peanuts)
2. dietary restrictions?	→	gluten intolerant (bread)
3. religious restrictions?	→	Jehovah's witness (blood transfusion)
4. religious restrictions?	→	Islamic (halal food)

● **Informing the Patient before an action**

P: I'm sorry. <u>I've wet the bed.</u>

N: Okay. I'm going to <u>change your sheets</u> for you.

....

P		N
1. "The room is getting dark."	→	turn on the lights
2. "I feel cramped."	→	move your pillow
3. "My legs feel uncomfortable."	→	raise the knee rest

> ■■■ **Communication Strategy** ■■■
> –Keep the patient informed–
>
> Foreign patients who need to have surgery in Japan, are often very anxious for what will happen to them. One reason for this is the language barrier. Another is that they don't know the detail of their surgeries. Always *keep your patient informed*. Explain the action, or ask about it, before you do something to the patient. （手術の前後は患者さ んは不安が多くなります。何かを行う際には必ず事前に説明するようにしましょう。）
>
> Use expressions like:
>
> ☐ I'm going to ~.
> ☐ Would you like me to ~?
> ☐ You need to have ~.
> ☐ The doctor will see you shortly.

WRITING PRACTICE 1

Form questions that you would ask before the following actions. Use "Would you like me to 〜 ?"

1) カーテンを閉める前：

_____.

2) 患者の背中を拭く前：

_____.

3) ベッドの頭を上げる前：

_____.

4) 枕を動かす前：

_____.

5) 患者の入れ歯を洗ってあげる前：

_____.

WRITING PRACTICE 2

Try to name as many objects as you can.

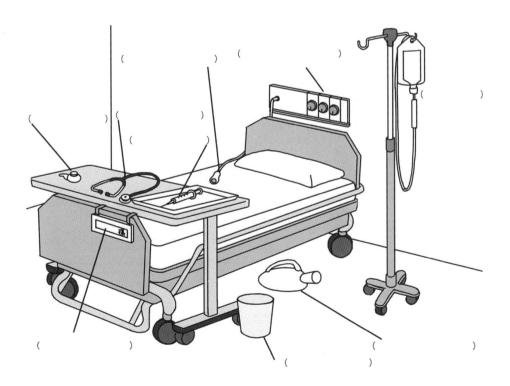

Unit 12   Are you feeling more comfortable now?

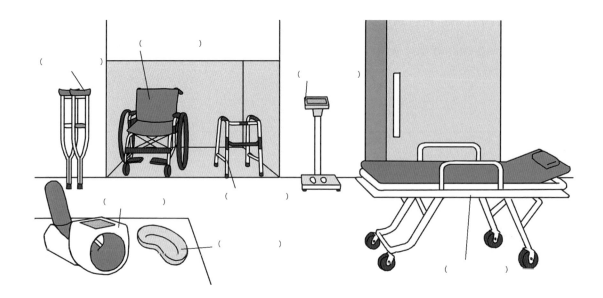

MEDICAL VOCABULARY

– Items around the Patient in the Hospital Room and Ward –

bandage	包帯	scale	はかり
band aid	バンドエイド	sling	つり包帯
bedpan	差し込み便器	sphygmomanometer	血圧計
bed rails	ベッドレール	spouted water cup	吸飲み
bedside cabinet	ベッドサイドキャビネット	stethoscope	聴診器
crutches	松葉杖	stretcher / gurney	ストレッチャー
emesis basin	膿盆	surgical tray	(処置) トレー
dressing (gauze)	ガーゼ	syringe	注射器
IV (intravenous) drip	点滴	thermometer	体温計
kidney basin	膿盆	tourniquet	止血帯
medical chart	カルテ	urinal	尿瓶
nurse call button	ナースコールボタン	walker	歩行器
overbed table	ベッドサイドテーブル	waste paper basket	紙屑 (ごみ) 箱
oxygen	酸素	wheelchair	車椅子

Cultural Quip

In Japan you call metal basins 膿盆 , and plastic basins ガーグルベースン , but in English there is, generally, no differentiation. Just say: metal (or plastic) kidney (or emesis) basin.

WORD POWER

AFFIX	MEANING	EXAMPLES
plac	静か	placebo, placid, complacency, placate
sens	感触	sensitive, consent, sensory, hypersensitivity
vita / viv	生命	vital signs, vitamins, revitalize, revive
trans	横切る	transplant, transfusion, translate, transverse colon
vid / vis	みる	review, supervise, visual, provide, vision

WRITING PRACTICE 3

Using the information about the Greek and Latin roots above, complete the exercise.

1. ____ We may be able to <u>transfer</u> the patient from the Recovery Room to his own room tomorrow.

2. ____ Normal <u>vital</u> signs figures change with age, sex, weight, and exercise.

3. ____ There was no <u>evidence</u> of scarring within the stomach.

4. ____ Mrs. Bryant felt better after she was given a <u>placebo</u>.

5. ____ Henry was very <u>sensitive</u> to sunlight, and spent most days indoors.

....

a. life

b. medicine used to quiet or calm rather than cure the patient

c. have strong feelings

d. move across from one place to another

e. something clearly seen, proof

Mini-Dictionary:

● recovery　回復

● scarring　傷跡

● calm　静める

DIALOGUE 12

First, listen to the recording. Then listen again, and fill in the blanks.

N: Good evening, Mr. Peters.

P: Hello, Nurse.

N: (1)_____? Nurse Miyake told me that you had a bad day.

P: Hmm.

N: Are you (2)_____?

P: Not really.

N: Well, yes. It looks like you've been sliding down the bed. Let me (3)_____.

P: Umph.

N: I'm going to (4)_____.

P: That feels better.

N: I'll leave the controller within your reach. Now, can I do anything else for you?

P: (5)_____.

N: Oh? That's no good. Let me see. This cover is a bit heavy. I'm going to (6)_____ and a blanket.

P: Thank you. At last someone is looking after me!

N: Oh, we all want to look after you. All you need to do is (7)_____.

P: Can I have a cup of tea?

N: I'll see (8)_____.

P: You know, when I was a pilot, the stewardess would always bring me round an extra cup of tea.

N: Oh? (9)_____ a pilot?

P: Yes. And I have some good stories to tell about my experiences!

N: Really? I'd love to hear some, but now (10)_____ some extra bedding.

Unit 13　This is an emergency.

Nurses always have to be prepared for the unexpected: not only medical emergencies, but also fires, explosions, earthquakes, weather-related crisis, and hazardous-substance releases.（看護師はいつも救急医療だけでなく災害などの想定外の出来事に出会う可能性があります。看護師としてそうした事態への心構えをしておきましょう。）

KEY EXPRESSIONS

NURSES' KEY EXPRESSIONS

1. James, can you hear me?
   「ジェームズ、聞こえますか？」
2. Can you explain what happened?
   「何が起こったのか説明できますか？」
3. Do you know where you are?
   「ここがどこなのかわかりますか？」
4. Can you move your fingers?
   「指を動かすことはできますか？」

■■■ Communication Strategy ■■■
–Make suggestions–

A patient may be under a lot of stress, and may not know how best to explain her problem. *Make suggestions*. （十分な情報を伝えることが出来ない患者さんに提案をしてあげてください。）

For example:

P: My shoulder hurts.
N: Can you describe the pain?
P: ......
N: Is it a sharp pain?
P: No.
N: Is it dull pain?
P: Yes. It's a dull pain.

WRITING PRACTICE 1

Label as many internal organs as you can and then check your answers with the list on the next page.

CENTRAL NERVOUS SYSTEM

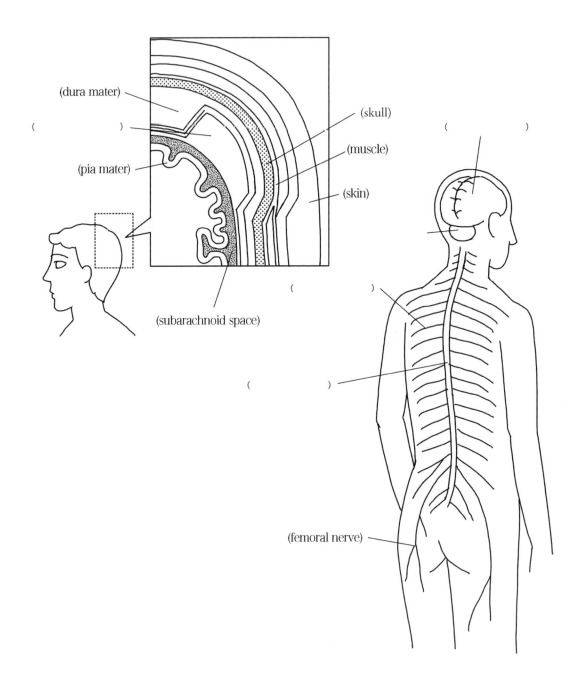

(dura mater)

(skull)

(   )

(   )

(muscle)

(pia mater)

(skin)

(   )

(subarachnoid space)

(   )

(femoral nerve)

CARDIOVASCULAR SYSTEM

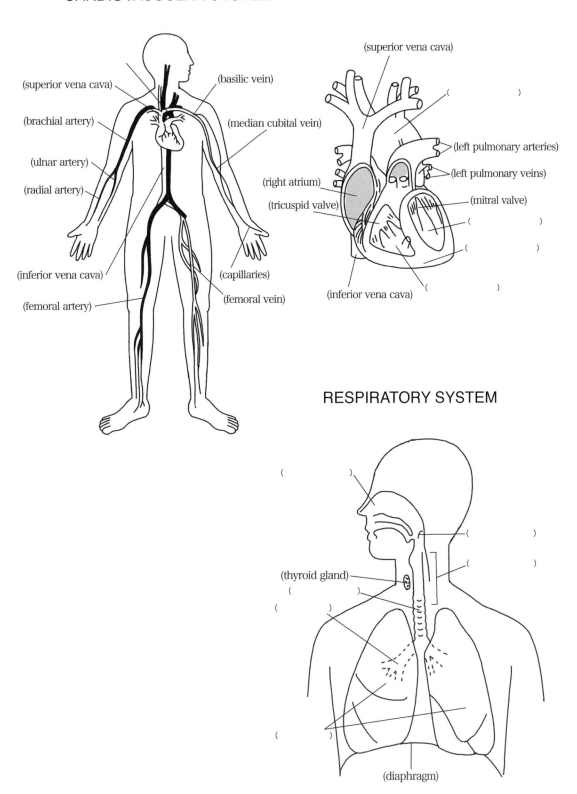

(superior vena cava)

(basilic vein)

(superior vena cava)

(brachial artery)

(median cubital vein)

(ulnar artery)

(radial artery)

(right atrium)

(tricuspid valve)

(left pulmonary arteries)

(left pulmonary veins)

(mitral valve)

(   )

(   )

(inferior vena cava)

(capillaries)

(femoral artery)

(femoral vein)

(inferior vena cava)

(   )

RESPIRATORY SYSTEM

(   )

(   )

(   )

(thyroid gland)

(   )

(   )

(   )

(diaphragm)

MEDICAL VOCABULARY
– Internal Organs (1) –

● CARDIOVASCULAR SYSTEM

arteries	動脈	left/right ventricle	左／右心室
atrium	心房	myocardium	心筋層
capillaries	毛細血管	valve	弁
heart	心臓	aorta	大動脈
veins	静脈		

● CENTRAL NERVOUS SYSTEM   ● RESPIRATORY SYSTEM

arachnoid	くも膜	bronchi	気管支
brain	脳	larynx	喉頭
cerebellum	小脳	lung	肺
cerebrum	大脳	nasal cavity	鼻
nerves	神経	pharynx	咽頭
spinal cord	脊髄	trachea	気管

MEDICAL VOCABULARY
– Emergencies –

● ACCIDENT CASES   ● MEDICAL CASES

abrasion	擦過創	cardiac arrest	心停止
bleeding	出血	cerebral hemorrhage	脳出血
bone fracture	骨折	cerebral infarction	脳梗塞
bruising	打撲	coronary thrombosis	冠動脈血栓症
burns	火傷・熱傷	dehydration	脱水症
car crash	交通事故	(epileptic) fit / seizure	（てんかん性）発作
cuts	切創	food poisoning	食中毒
drowned	溺死	heart attack	心臓発作
drowning	溺水	heat stress disorder	熱中症
fall	落下	heat stroke / sun stroke	熱射病・日射病
lacerations	裂創	hypoxia	低酸素
poisoning	中毒	myocardial infarction	心筋梗塞
puncture	刺創	pneumothorax / collapsed lung	気胸症
suffocation	窒息	stroke	脳卒中
water accident	水の事故	unconscious	意識がない
whiplash	むち打ち	vomiting	嘔吐

SPEAKING PRACTICE 1

Practice the following conversation with a partner and continue with the substitution drills, or make your own. （ICU に入ってくる患者さんの状態について説明する練習をしましょう。）

N1: What happened?

N2: <u>The patient was in a car crash</u>.

N1: And what is his (her) condition?

N2: <u>He has multiple fractures</u>.

1. This child was in a water accident. He nearly drowned. /
   He has water in his lungs.

2. The patient was in a *light aircraft accident. /
   He has second degree burns to 30 % of his body.

3. This man fell off a ladder. /
   He has a punctured lung.

4. The patient was admitted with a collapsed lung. /
   She is suffering from hypoxia.

5. This woman fell from a horse. /
   She has a damaged spinal cord.

6. The patient has deep cuts. /
   She is bleeding heavily.

7. The patient was in a *hazardous-substance accident. /
   He is vomiting.

8. The patient was hit by *flying objects in the typhoon. /
   He is unconscious.

Mini-Dictionary:
- light aircraft　軽飛行機
- hazardous-substance　有害物質
  ≒ hazardous household chemicals:（家庭にある）有害化合品；例えば、塩素、防虫剤、電池など
- flying objects　飛来物

WRITING PRACTICE 2

Match the illnesses with some symptoms or causes. （以下の病名とそれに伴う症状を線で結んで下さい。）

<u>The illness</u>

1. cerebral hemorrhage •
2. tonsillitis •
3. myocardial infarction •
4. sun stroke •
5. hives •
6. meningitis •

<u>Possible symptoms</u>

• a. fever, headache, stiff neck, and decreased consciousness

• b. fever, pain when swallowing, inflamed tonsils

• c. redness, swelling, and itching of skin caused by an allergic reaction

• d. loss of consciousness, abrupt severe headache, bleeding within the brain

• e. crushing pain in the chest, death of part of the heart

• f. a red face, nausea, and difficulty breathing

WORD POWER

AFFIX	MEANING	EXAMPLES
sci	知識	conscious, unconscious, conscience
mort	死	mortuary, mortality rate, postmortem
rupt	破裂	rupture, interrupt, disrupt, skin eruption
hydro	水	dehydration, hydrotherapy, hydrocephalic
bio	生命	biological parents, biopsy, biotechnology

WRITING PRACTICE 3

Using the information about the Greek and Latin roots above, complete the exercise.

1. ___ Mary was <u>unconscious</u> when she entered hospital.
2. ___ The <u>biopsy</u> of the tissue from the tumor showed that it was benign.
3. ___ The patient suffered from <u>hydrothorax</u>.
4. ___ The accident patient arrived with a <u>ruptured</u> spleen.
5. ___ During the armed robbery the shop owner received a <u>mortal</u> wound.

....

  a. fluid (water) in the chest / lung
  b. not knowing what is happening around oneself
  c. deadly
  d. an examination of a small piece of living tissue
  e. something broken or torn

Mini-Dictionary:

● tissue　細胞の組織   ● spleen　脾臓

DIALOGUE 13

First, listen to the recording. Then listen again, and fill in the blanks.

N: Hello. Your name is?

EB: Elizabeth Borrows.

N: And this is?

EB: Leo Cliff.

N: Are you (1)_____ the patient?

EB: No.

N: Can you (2)_____ then?

EB: We were in class, giving our self-introductions in Japanese ...

N: At the university?

EB: Yes. Leo had just finished his speech and had sat down when he (3)_____ and fell on the floor.

N: And you knew he was having (4)_____?

EB: Well, yeah!

N: So what did you do?

EB: Well, we lay him down on his side. Gave him room to breathe. I made sure he didn't bite his tongue. You know ... checked that his (5)_____.

N: And how long was he like that?

EB: Not so long. Someone (6)_____ straight away.

N: I mean how long did the seizure last?

EB: Gosh. I'm not sure. Maybe 10 minutes. He (7)_____ while we were in the ambulance.

N: And is he (8)_____.

EB: I don't know.

N: How long have you known the patient?

EB: Only a couple of days. We came out together from Sydney.

N: And (9)_____ he's had a seizure?

EB: I don't know. I come from Tasmania, you know, the southern end of Australia, and he's from the north. We met on the plane.

N: And do you know if he is taking any medication?

EB: I know he takes some tablets in the morning and some at night. But I don't know what.

N: Okay. We'll (10)_____ and a record of his medication. I expect he has Health Insurance.

EB: Yeah, we all have Travel Insurance. I'll ask his host Mum to bring in his papers.

Unit 14　Tests show you have high sugar levels.

WARM-UP

The Full Medical Examination is known in Japan as 人間ドック. This term comes from the word for human（人間）and the ship being in dock（ドック）for safety checks and repairs. Do you know what tests are done at this time?（患者さんが人間ドックに入っている時、どのような検査をしているのでしょうか。）

KEY EXPRESSIONS

> **NURSES' KEY EXPRESSIONS**
>
> 1. Please change into these pajamas.
>   「パジャマに着替えてください」
> 2. We need to do an EEG and an ECG.
>   「脳波と心電図の検査をする必要があります」
> 3. Is there anything about your health that you are worried about?
>   「健康面で心配している事はありますか？」
> 4. I will tell the doctor your wish to know more about the test.
>   「検査についてお知りになりたいことがある旨を先生に伝えます」
> 5. Cholesterol levels can be checked with a simple blood test.
>   「コレステロール値を簡単な血液検査でチェックできます」

> **PATIENTS' KEY EXPRESSIONS**
>
> 1. I'd like the doctor to explain the results of the blood test.
>   「血液検査の結果を先生に説明していただきたいです」
> 2. I'd like some advice on how to lose weight.
>   「体重の減らし方についてアドバイスが欲しいです」

■■■ Communication Strategy ■■■
–Open-ended questions–

Interact with your patient. By asking *open-ended questions*, you give
the patient a chance to expand on how they are feeling. （自由に解答できる
質問をすると、患者さんがもっと親身になって語ってくれる可能性があります。）

For example:
Can you tell me more?
And how did the medication work for you?
How do these symptoms affect your everyday life?

WRITING PRACTICE 1

Label as many internal organs as you can and then check your answers with
the list on the next page.

ORAL CAVITY

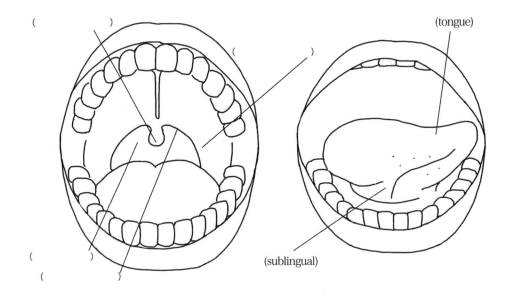

DIGESTIVE SYSTEM

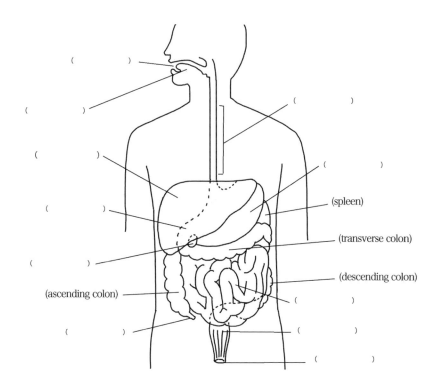

(   )

(   )

(   )

(   )

(   )

(ascending colon)

(   )

(   )

(spleen)

(transverse colon)

(descending colon)

(   )

(   )

(   )

UROGENITAL SYSTEM

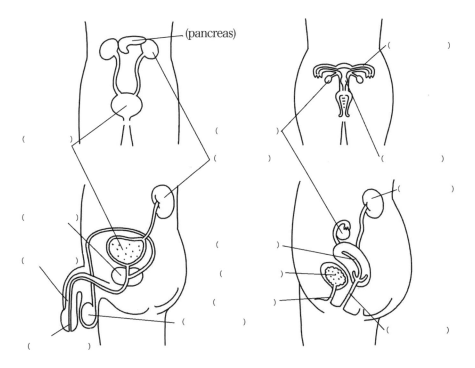

(pancreas)

(   )

(   )

(   )

(   )

(   )

(   )

(   )

(   )

(   )

(   )

(   )

(   )

(   )

(   )

Unit 14   Tests show you have high sugar levels.

MEDICAL VOCABULARY
– Internal Organs (2) –

● ORAL CAVITY

adenoids	腺様
throat	のど
tonsils	扁桃
uvula	垂

● DIGESTIVE SYSTEM

anus	肛門
appendix	盲腸・虫垂
colon	結腸
duodenum	十二指腸
esophagus	食道
gallbladder	胆嚢
large intestine	大腸
liver	肝臓
oral cavity	口
rectum	直腸
small intestine	小腸
stomach	胃
(sublingual) salivary gland	（舌下）唾腺

● UROGENITAL SYSTEM

bladder	膀胱
fallopian tube	卵管
kidneys	腎臓
ovary	卵巣
penis	陰茎
prostate gland	前立腺
testicle	睾丸
urethra	尿道
uterus (womb)	子宮
vagina	膣

● UROGENITAL SYSTEM

pancreas	膵臓
spleen	脾臓
thyroid gland	甲状腺

MEDICAL VOCABULARY
– Medical Tests –

● GENERAL TESTS

blood test	血液検査	lung function test	肺機能検査
chest X-ray	胸のレントゲン	sputum test	喀痰検査
ECG (Electrocardiogram)	心電図	stool test	検便
EEG (Electroencephalogram)	脳波	ultrasound (echogram)	超音波検査
visual acuity test	視力検査	Doppler ultrasound	ドップラー超音波検査
hearing (audiometry) test	聴力検査	urinalysis	尿検査

● SPECIALIZED TESTS

bronchoscopy	気管支鏡検査	gastroscopy	胃内視鏡検査
colonoscopy	大腸内視鏡検査	laparoscopy	腹腔鏡検査
cystoscopy	膀胱鏡検査	spinal tap	腰椎穿刺
endoscopy	内視鏡検査	thermography	サーモグラフィー

BMD (Bone Mineral Density) Test　骨塩密度：骨塩定量測定検査（骨密度検査）

CT (CAT) scan (Computerized Axial Tomography)　コンピュータ断層撮影

MRI (Magnetic Resonance Imaging)　磁気共鳴映像法

upper GI series (barium meal)　上部消化器造影（バリウム粥）

lower GI series (barium enema)　下部消化器造影（バリウム注腸）

mammogram　乳房造影図（マンモグラム）

Pap test　パップ試験（子宮癌検査法）(uterine cancer screening)

Reference

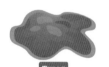

Type 7
Liquid consistency with no solid pieces
(Severe diarrhea)

Type 1
Separate hard lumps
(Severe constipation)

Type 6
Mushy consistency
with ragged edges
(Mild diarrhea)

BRISTOL STOOL CHART

Type 2
Lumpy and sausage-like
(Mild constipation)

Type 5
Soft blobs with clear-cut edges
(Lacking fiber)

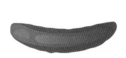

Type 4
Like a smooth soft sausage or snake
(Normal)

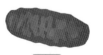

Type 3
Sausage shape with cracks
(Normal)

Unit 14　Tests show you have high sugar levels.

SPEAKING PRACTICE 1

Practice the dialogue with a partner and then expand with the substitution drills. (患者を検査に導く会話を練習しましょう。)

N: We need to do <u>an ECG</u>. Please <u>lie down here</u>.

P: Okay.

....

1. a hearing test.   / go to that room.

2. an ultrasound.   / bend your knees.

3. a chest X-ray.   / stand up here and turn this way.

4. a lung function test.   / put your mouth over this mouthpiece and
                             breathe in.

5. a bone density test.   / go to Radiology, Window 35.

WRITING PRACTICE 2

Write out an explanation of the test for the patient.

eg. cystoscopy   <u>An examination of the lining of the bladder
                        and the urethra.</u>

1. a fetal ultrasound   _____.

2. an audiometry test   _____.

3. a BMD   _____.

4. an upper endoscopy   _____.

5. an EEG   _____.

6. an upper GI series   _____.

7. a colonoscopy   _____.

8. a mammogram   _____.

WORD POWER

AFFIX	MEANING	EXAMPLES
scope / scopy	鏡	microscope, endoscopy, laparoscopy
osis	状態	neurosis, adiposis, osteoporosis
reg / rect	正、直	rectum, rectify, regulate, correct
gram / graph	書く・描く	electrocardiogram, diagram, biography
ultra	超・超えた	ultrasound, ultraviolet rays, ultimate

WRITING PRACTICE 3

Using the information about the Greek and Latin roots above, complete the exercise.

1. ____ After the epileptic fit, she came in regularly for an electroencephalogram (EEG).

2. ____ Sitting for long periods of time, like on a long plane trip, can result in <u>thrombosis</u>.

3. ____ Joanne began to <u>rectify</u> her weight problem by starting a daily exercise routine.

4. ____ In order to cut <u>ultraviolet</u> rays, we should use parasols, or wide brimmed hats.

5. ____ It is very important to thoroughly clean out the colon before a <u>colonoscopy</u>.

....

   a. an examination of the inside of the colon
   b. beyond the purple in the visible light range
   c. the state of having blood clots
   d. to set straight / to correct errors
   e. a chart of the electric impulses of the brain

Mini-Dictionary:

● routine　日課・通常の　　　　　　● parasol　日傘

DIALOGUE 14

First, listen to the recording. Then listen again, and fill in the blanks.

N: Mrs. Suzuki-Crowe?

P: Yes?

N: You're here to hear a report (1)_____?

P: Yes.

N: Is there (2)_____ about your health that you are worried about and want to ask the doctor?

P: Well, first I want the doctor to (3)_____ of the blood test.

N: I see.

P: I'm always a little anemic, and I want to know why, and what I should do about it.

N: Good. Anything else?

P: Yes. I had both a mammogram and (4)_____ on my breast. I know I have a lump there. How would they do a biopsy if the doctor suggests it?

N: They put a fine needle into the lump and draw out (5)_____ _____.

P: Oh? Is it dangerous? Do I really need it?

N: It's not dangerous. But I will tell the doctor your wish to know more about it.

P: I also drank that awful barium stuff, right?

N: Yes. You took (6)_____ tests.

P: Well I often get (7)_____, and I was wondering if anything came up in the tests.

N: Okay.

P: Did I forget something?

N: Your tests show that you have (8)_____. Perhaps you would like to ask the doctor about that.

P: Diabetes? Oh! I hope not! But I do want to know about how to bring down my cholesterol levels.

N: You have (9)_____, don't you, Mrs. Suzuki?

P: Yes. I'm at the desk all day.

N: A lack of exercise and carrying extra weight can be (10)_____
_____.

P: Yeah. Just tell the doctor I want to ask lots of questions.

Unit 15   You'll be leaving us soon.

Ideally, the patient is being discharged because they have gotten over the worst of their illness and are now on the road to recovery. Being transferred to a tertiary care facility, a hospital closer to the patient's home, or to a hospice facility may also be a reason for leaving. Although mostly an administrative procedure, the nurse should still give care and help the patient or direct family till the very end of the stay, perhaps giving advice towards the next step.

There is, of course, the death of the client. In the case of a client who had been visiting from overseas, this can be a more complicated procedure as the Embassy will also need to be contacted.

(患者さんの退院は、病気の峠を越し改善・完治に向かっている状態がベストですが、時には、より高度な医療施設へ転院や、地域の病院へ戻ることや、ホスピスへ入ることなどの理由で退院することもあります。そして、患者さんがお亡くなりになったため「退院」するということもあります。その際、海外からの短期滞在者である場合、手続きが複雑になる可能性があります。)

KEY EXPRESSIONS

NURSES' KEY EXPRESSIONS

1. I hear you'll be going home soon.
   「もうすぐ帰宅されると伺いました」
2. Don't forget to monitor your blood pressure every day.
   「毎日血圧を測る事を忘れないでください」
3. You should bathe the baby during the day when it's warmer.
   「日中の暖かい時に赤ちゃんを入浴させましょう」
4. Take this invoice downstairs to the accounts department and pay there. 「この請求書を持って下の階の会計課に行き、そこでお支払いください」

PATIENTS' KEY EXPRESSIONS

1. I want to get full copies of my medical records from here.
   「ここで受けた治療記録の全ての写しが欲しいです」
2. I want to know about follow-up care.
   「追加の治療について知りたいです」
3. I know I'm dying. Can someone talk to me about Hospice?
   「死が近づいていることがわかります。ホスピスについてお話できる人はいますか？」

> ### ■■■ Communication Strategy ■■■
> –Encourage your patient–
>
> Even when the figures say that the situation is not getting better, try to keep positive, and caring. （患者さんの容態や検査の数字がよくならないときでも、患者さんを励ましたり、温和な態度で接したりして下さい。）
>
> > For example:
> >
> > You've been doing well.
> >
> > I know you'll be able to manage.
> >
> > Thank you for being such a good patient.
> >
> > You need to continue your rehabilitation exercises at home.

SPEAKING PRACTICE 1 (INCLUDING FOR A DYING PATIENT)

Here are some patient comments. Think of your own comments or use the hints to make an answer for the patient. （患者さんからの一言に対してどう対応しますか？ヒントを活用し、自分のコメントを考えて答えてください。）

Example:

P: "This is so embarrassing. I can't even go to the toilet by myself."

→ N: Don't worry Hank. We are just paying you back for all the help you gave us when we were young.

---

1. "The pain is getting worse."
   → 痛みの詳しい説明 （where? describe the pain? different to other pain?）

2. "I'm sorry if my family is being loud when they come."
   → 個室 （private room?）

3. "I think I'm going to die." （冗談半分・少し心細時に）
   → まだ （not yet）

4. "Am I really going to die?" （末期がんの患者に）
   → 自然の歩み （everyone, life's journey）

5. "I'm so sorry to be a burden."
   → 模範な患者 （good patient, not a burden, our job）

Unit 15   You'll be leaving us soon.

WRITING PRACTICE 1

Choose from the list below, which category the patient would belong to.
（下記のリストから患者さんがどのカテゴリに入るか考え、選びなさい。）

The American Society of Anesthesiologists (ASA) Physical Status Classification System

Classification	Definition	Examples	答え
ASA I	A normal, healthy patient	The patient doesn't smoke or drink.	
ASA II	A patient with a mild systemic disease that does not limit activity	The patient is a smoker. The patient is pregnant. The patient is a social drinker. The patient has a history of dysrhythmia controlled on medication.	
ASA III	A patient with a severe systemic disease	The patient has poorly controlled diabetes. The patient's BMI is over 40 (morbid obesity). The patient has hepatitis.	
ASA IV	A patient with a severe systemic disease that is a constant threat to his or her life	The patient has end-stage renal disease. The patient has ongoing cardiac ischemia. The patient has malignant hypertension.	
ASA V	A moribund patient who is not expected to survive 24 hours without surgery	The patient has intracranial bleeding. The patient has congestive heart failure (CHF). The patient has been in a traumatic traffic accident.	
ASA VI	A patient who has been declared brain dead and whose organs can be removed for donation		

a) 脳死と判断された患者で、臓器提供を明記した者。
b) 大動脈瘤が破裂し、運ばれた者。
c) 喘息を患っている者
d) 遡って、3か月以内に心筋梗塞（MI）を経験した者。
e) 血圧が 115/75 で、健康な者。
f) ペースメーカを植え込まれた者

WRITING PRACTICE 2

Read the Letter and check the content of each category. （紹介状を読んで、下記の項目毎に状況を記入してください。）

Letter of Referral

<u>Name</u>: Mr. George SMITH   <u>Sex</u>: Male   <u>D.O.B.</u>: 13-08-1960
<u>Nationality</u>: British   <u>Address in Japan</u>: Peacock Hotel, Osaka

<u>History of Presenting Complaint</u>:
Mr. Smith presented with lower back pain on the left side and the need to urinate frequently. An ultrasound and contrast-enhanced CT showed a simple kidney cyst. Classified as Bosniak IIF Cyst >3cm diameter. The cyst was aspirated and sclerotherapy done.
No further investigations have been performed or requested.

<u>Reason for Referral</u>:
I would appreciate it if Mr. Smith's status could be reevaluated through a follow-up ultrasound and observation after his return to his homeland.

1. 病院を訪れた理由：＿＿＿＿＿＿＿＿＿＿＿＿＿＿＿＿＿＿＿＿＿＿＿＿＿

2. 検査の結果：＿＿＿＿＿＿＿＿＿＿＿＿＿＿＿＿＿＿＿＿＿＿＿＿＿＿＿

3. 治療方法：＿＿＿＿＿＿＿＿＿＿＿＿＿＿＿＿＿＿＿＿＿＿＿＿＿＿＿＿

4. 帰国後：＿＿＿＿＿＿＿＿＿＿＿＿＿＿＿＿＿＿＿＿＿＿＿＿＿＿＿＿＿

SPEAKING PRACTICE 2

 Match the category with some symptoms or causes.（退院時に確認する項目と表現を線で結んで下さい。）

Hospital Discharge Checklist （退院時のチェックリスト）

項目	表現

1. Medication •

2. Medical insurance form •

3. X-rays •

4. Personal belongings •

5. Diet program •

6. Exercise routine •

7. Discharge summary •
   (Letter of Referral)

8. Contact information •

9. Follow-up appointments •

• a. Do you have everything? Nothing forgotten?

• b. Copies of your x-rays and MRI are on this disk. Please give it to your family doctor.

• c. A dietician will come to see you soon to talk about your diet.

• d. Here is your medication. Please continue as directed.

• e. The doctor has filled in your travel insurance form.

• f. This shows the date of your next checkup, in a year's time.

• g. Here is the file showing your home exercise routine.

• h. This is your Letter of Referral describing your treatment here.

• i. This shows who you can contact if you have any questions.

 # WORD POWER

AFFIX	MEANING	EXAMPLES
meter	測り	glucometer, sphygmomanometer, spirometer, oximeter
vert	回転する	vertebra, vertigo, vertex, vertical
sa / sat	満たす	saturate, satisfaction, satiate, polyunsaturated
tain	保つ	retain, container, abstain, maintain
flex	曲げる	flexible, flexion, reflexes, flexor

WRITING PRACTICE 3

Study the affixes in the Word Power list and match the meanings with the words underlined in the sentences below. （上記の語源のリストを見て、下記の文章中の下線の言葉の意味を a ～ e から探しなさい。）

1. ＿＿ A <u>spirometer</u> is the main piece of equipment used for basic Pulmonary Function tests.

2. ＿＿ An x-ray of the cervical <u>vertebrae</u> showed that there was pressure on the C6 nerve root.

3. ＿＿ Some patients were <u>dissatisfied</u> with the health care services they received there.

4. ＿＿ In spite of being in a serious accident, he <u>sustain</u>ed only light injuries.

5. ＿＿ Newborn babies have several reflexes not in adults, such as the grasp <u>reflex</u>.

....

    a. a muscle movement in response to a stimulus

    b. small bones that make up the spine, allowing us to turn about

    c. a machine for measuring the volume of air inspired and expired by the lungs

    d. not feeling happy or fulfilled

    e. to suffer; to endure; to experience something bad

Mini-Dictionary:

● Pulmonary Function test　肺機能検査

DIALOGUE 15

First, listen to the recording. Then listen again, and fill in the blanks.

Going home with baby

N: Well, Mr. and Mrs. Brown, I'm sure (1)_____ to be going home this afternoon.

B: Yes, but I'm also wondering if we will be able to (2)_____ _____ by ourselves.

N: Well, today you'll be given the job of (3)_____, not just watching us like yesterday.

B: Yes. I've prepared some clothes here for him to wear afterwards.

N: Okay. Before you put the baby in the bath, make sure the room is warm. Undress him and lay a gauze towel (4)_____ covering his hands.

B: Why over his hands?

N: To give a sense of comfort. After being in (5)_____ for nine months, the baby can get surprised at so much freedom.

B: How should I hold his head? Should I rest it on my arm?

N: That (6)_____. Hold his head in the palm of your hand. Put your thumb over one ear and your (7)_____ over the other.

B: I noticed last time that you put something in the bath already. Do you always do that? Can I use a mild soap at home?

N: A new-born isn't really dirty, and some soaps are too strong for a baby's (8)_____.

B: I'll follow the recommendations then.

N: And to wash his back…

B: I know. I flip him over. I slide my hand under his armpit and lay his head on my arm. It's like (9)_____.

N: You're doing well. I know (10)_____ him well after you get home.

学生の皆さんに
― あとがきにかえて ―

　昔々、笑顔のとっても可愛い女の子がいました。お兄ちゃんと遊ぶのがとても好きで、生まれたばかりの妹の世話をするのも大好きでした。しかし、2歳のある夏の日、彼女の笑顔は突然消えてしまいました。

　彼女の脳に、ウイルスが忍び込んだのです。

　髄膜炎とされた次の日には脳炎であると診断されました。意識不明の状態が一週間続いた後、ようやく意識が戻りました。容態は少しよくなりましたが、すぐまた悪化しました。それから大きな発作が1回あり、医師から「一生寝たきり」と診断される重い障害を負うことになりました。

　半年間にも及ぶ入院の初めの頃、発作によって後遺症が残った彼女を療法士たちは避けがちでした。病室の前を通るナースたちは声をひそめ、面会には誰も来ませんでした。毎日徹夜で看護するその子の母親に、自分たちはどのように接すればいいのか、彼らにはわからなかったのです。お母さんはいつも「英語」で子どもに話しかけていました。当時は英語を理解できる看護師は少なく、英語でどんな言葉を二人にかければいいのか、見当もつかなかったのでしょう。

　そのような状況にあっても、お母さんは毎日その子に話しかけ、いつか目が見えるようになるかもしれない時のために絵を描きました。筋肉が元の柔軟性を取り戻すように、子供の腕と足を一生懸命さすり続けました。

　あの出来事から30年以上の歳月が流れ、彼女はすっかり成長しました。ハンディはあるものの、一生寝たきりではありません。そして何よりも、あの時の可愛らしい笑顔が戻りました。

　学生の皆さんにお願いがあります。慣れない言語で医療を学んでいると、挫折しそうになることもあるかもしれません。でも、そんな時には、この脳炎になった子のことを思い出して欲しいのです。あの時、彼女自身も含めてみんなが「できない」とか「もうだめ」と思ったら、彼女は成人式を迎えることはなかったでしょうし、今こうして笑顔に溢れた生活をおくることも出来なかったと思うのです。

　最初は看護師の励まし、それから後に療法士の励ましが、彼女を、私の娘を「できない子」から少しずつ「できる子」に育てたのです。

　学生の皆さんもこれから関わる患者さんに笑顔が戻ってくるように接してあげてください。国籍・言葉は関係なしに。言葉のうまく通じない国で不安を沢山抱えた彼らが最も必要としているものは、あなた方の心からの優しさなのです。

山中

看護系学生のための実践英語 ［改訂版］

| 検印省略 | ©2021 年 1 月 31 日　　初版発行
2023 年 1 月 31 日　　第 3 刷発行 |

編著者　　　　　　　　　　　　　山中マーガレット
発行者　　　　　　　　　　　　　原　　雅久
発売所　　　　　　　　　　株式会社 朝日出版社

101-0065　東京都千代田区西神田 3-3-5
電話（03）3239-0271
FAX（03）3239-0479
e-mail: text-e@asahipress.com
振替口座　00140-2-46008
組版・Office haru ／製版・錦明印刷

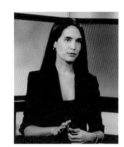
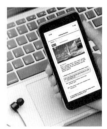